The Manual

Vol. 6

Central Virginia Sport Performance

The sixth collaboration of works from our contributors

The Manual

Vol. 6

Central Virginia Sport Performance

Edited By:
Jay DeMayo, CSCS
Andrew White, MS, CSCS
Mike Thomson, MS, CSCS

Published by: Central Virginia Sport Performance, Richmond VA 23238
For information and to order copies: www.cvasps.com

Table of Contents

Forward

This year has been hard.

I think that is a statement that we have all uttered repeatedly while undergoing massive amounts of testing, going on pauses, revaluating how the restarting procedure "should" go, constant stress and fear of what may come from the next test results, and the constant feeling of turning blind corners every day. The past year has brought out so many different emotions. From the joy of returning to the gym and having the teams return, to the fear of the unknown with everything associated with living and working through a pandemic, to the trauma you would see from people who were "locked up" in quarantine. Each and every aspect of it was hard, but with the hard came a lot of learning and reflecting. For each situation that popped up that brought worry about the daily lives of those in our profession it sparked a new question:

- When I saw those who were unfortunate enough to lose their jobs it made me question my savings habits and how I handle the money I was making at that point.
- Seeing those go through the stress of a furlough made me ask if the additional work I do outside the school would be enough for me to keep the lights on, and if not, needs to be done better.
- Looking at people who had the terrible circumstance of catching the virus and going through the worst of its symptoms made me look deeper into my health, fitness, nutrition, stress management, and sleep strategies.

It has been hard, but I hope some of the hard has helped you find your way to be in a better place. If you haven't found that better place yet, I hope that at the very least, it has helped you ask better questions to pursue ways to do just that.

I hope you enjoy The Manual, Vol. 6

Jay "Greybeard" DeMayo

1

Coloring Outside the Lines

Leading Authentically and Creating an Athlete Partnership

Molly Binneti

Take a moment to reflect internally, as a child you remember being in school and being given an image of something. Maybe it was something simple and boring, such as a house, or a picture of all the animals at the zoo, and you had to color the image with crayons. You had to – or you were instructed to – stay inside the lines of the image. Beyond that, you were expected to use the "right" colors; the grass had to be green, the sky had to be blue. Your teachers and Kindergarten friends noticed when your crayons strayed, or you used colors that did not match reality. Everyone knows the grass is not pink and the sky is not purple, even though in the moment YOU wanted to color them this way. Maybe you even got judged or made fun of if your image looked different than everybody else's.

We learn to color inside the lines in Kindergarten, as well as other things like; share everything, play fair, do not hit people, put things back where you found them, and look both ways before crossing the street. Guidelines that remain useful even in our adult lives...for the most part.

As we grow up, we are continuously being shaped and molded by the society we live in. We become conditioned by the people we surround ourselves with and the environment with which we spend the most time. Culture dictates the values, beliefs, and assumptions we adopt about ourselves and the world. The same rings true when we begin our journey as professionals and navigate the tumultuous world of strength and conditioning. Our education is centered around anatomy, physiology, biomechanics, exercise technique, program design, training adaptations and responses to exercise – the cornerstones of understanding the human body and improving athletic performance. Through our experiences shadowing, interning, and learning from those who came before us we get our first taste of what it means to be a strength coach – behaviors, coaching and leadership styles, stereotypes, and expectations.

Like we were taught to color inside the lines as a child, there are ways in which we are told to color inside the lines in our careers. Take a moment to reflect again; in what ways were you told how to be a strength coach or shown what it means to be a strength coach? To expand a little further, what were you told makes a leader or shown what qualities were required to exhibit leadership?

As a young coach, I spent the better part of my time being heavily influenced by the other coaches around me and trying to emulate them because I didn't know any better. We spend a tremendous amount of time learning what to coach. Many of us think a lot about WHY we coach. However, nothing really prepares us, and no one teaches us HOW to coach. I'm not talking about how to coach a squat or a clean. I'm talking about people. How to impact, empower, and connect with people to help them grow into the best version of themselves and accomplish the mission they desire for themselves. To be frank – I wasn't thinking about that in the early stages of my career. I was consumed with writing the best programs and coaching the best lift or speed sessions of all time, thinking that would equate to my success. Everything I learned about how to coach was through observation and I picked up tidbits on leadership, reading various generic books on the topic. Below is a thorough yet condensed list of what I was told to be true:

- …A dominant and controlling style is the most effective way to run a session or lead people.

- …Women have a hard time succeeding in this field because they don't command the same respect.

- …Bringing the "juice" is a job requirement.

- …Being a hype man or hype woman is a job requirement.

- …Perfection is always the goal. If it's not perfect, there is a consequence.

- …Athletes should be miserable when they are in the weight room.

- …Loud means you are effective.

- …Following rules = discipline.

- …Nobody likes an athlete who isn't compliant.

- …Fear tactics are most effective to get the desired behavior.

- …We are the coach – athletes should respect and trust us no matter what.

- …We are the experts and the decision makers; we know what is best for our athletes.

- …Show no weakness, stay in control.

What I was *taught* to be true and what I *felt* to be true was always at odds. I remember being in a state of cognitive dissonance as early as age 24, my second year as a full-time coach. Cognitive dissonance occurs when a person holds contradictory beliefs, ideas, or values, and experiences stress when he or she behaves in a way that goes against one or more of them. I questioned whether I was cut out for this field because I didn't feel like I could live up to the perception of how I was supposed to act. I felt a constant need to exude a certain persona that never felt natural. I felt continuously frustrated that my athletes were not buying in fully nor changing the behaviors that were detrimental to them.

All of this culminated in 2018 when I was 28 and about to venture into a high-profile new position. I had a chip on my shoulder, eager to prove my value and set the tone for the way I wanted things to be done. I was in charge and relished being in control for the first time in my career. While our athletes got healthier, stronger, and faster – we even made a Sweet 16 appearance – I was slowly burning the candle at both ends until I found myself completely burned out and in a constant state of tension. We had zero injuries that year, and all of our performance metrics improved – by most people's account of what it means to be a good strength coach, I was doing pretty well. However, most of my time was spent being a dictator and disciplining athletes who weren't following the rules. I felt like I had to be a hard-ass to get anything accomplished, which is not who I am at all. I was struggling to get them to change their behaviors and resorted to getting them to be obedient in the moment. My relationships with them were surface level. All of it felt overwhelming and frustrating. I was going to bed asking myself these questions:

1) What do I want MOST for myself and my athletes?

2) What am I trying to prove? And to whom?

3) What difference am I really making?

4) How are other people experiencing me?

5) What type of environment am I creating for my athletes?

The answers to these questions were unpleasant to sit with. The reality is, we rarely make a change until we hit rock bottom or close to it and we are forced to. I was miserable for a few reasons:

1) I was trying to be someone I'm not and coaching in a way completely inauthentic to who I am.

2) I spent most of my time getting our athletes to simply comply and follow rules.

3) Because of the above, I knew I was short-changing the amount of impact I had and the value I was bringing. The relationships I had with our athletes suffered.

4) I knew there was more. More learning, more connection, more impact, more development. There had to be a better way.

Cross · roads

/ krôs rōdz/
Noun
The point in which an important choice must be made.

Often, when we fail to get the results we want, it is second nature to look outside ourselves and point fingers towards the reasons things went wrong. It was easy for me to pass the blame for the lack of compliance buy-in towards the weight room, and mediocre relationships with the athletes and chalk it up to them being "difficult." It was true, they were being difficult, but when I truly reflected on the year and what needed to improve, I had to get real because...

All improvement starts with the truth.

The truth was this:

• ...All of my frustrations stemmed from relationships and elements of communication.

• ...I spent more time trying to manage the weight room and focusing on short-term results rather than building stronger connections with the people in front of me.

- …If my athletes weren't listening or learning, that is MY fault and responsibility, not theirs.

- …Reading another article, listening to another podcast, or attending another conference was not going to help me become a better person or leader.

- …I had to look long and hard into the mirror and point the finger back at myself.

- …Writing a better program was not going to move the needle. I had to be better.

We all love to take responsibility for our success and happiness. But taking responsibility for our problems is far more important. That is where real growth comes from. That is where real leadership comes from. When I think about my mission as a coach, it is to empower people to tell their championship stories. To equip them with the skills to not only understand and train their bodies, but also to ask questions, to solve problems, to take ownership, and to be able to navigate what life throws at them.

When I hit this crossroads my two choices were:

a.) Continue coloring inside the lines and coaching the way I was "expected" to

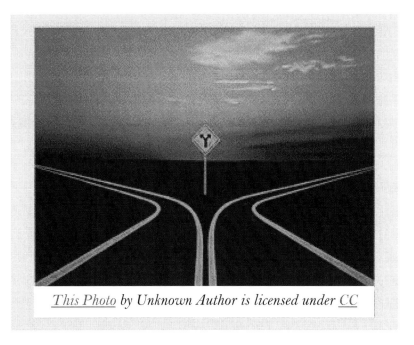

Have the courage to stray and try something different

One of the most difficult things we encounter as coaches is to relinquish control because it is in our nature. I prided myself on running the room and being the decision maker – I told and showed athletes what to do and they did it. The best way to describe that was a dictatorship. While I loved the control, it always felt inauthentic to me to play the role of the "tough guy" and disciplinarian. I'm not inherently loud and don't find it particularly enjoyable to yell in people's faces or punish them for a wrongdoing. I knew the only way to live and bring joy back to coaching was to be true to myself and harness the strengths of my personality to impact those around me. Rather than a dictatorship, I made the decision to go a different route and focus on creating an athlete partnership – establishing an environment and experience they took ownership of and that produced more intrinsic motivation. After all, the athlete's mission, the desirable future they want to achieve, is what matters most – not our agenda in the weight room or our ability to run a perfectly disciplined session.

To truly move the needle in my life and in the lives of the athletes I coach, it was not going to be achieved through designing a better training program or utilizing a piece of technology. It was going to be through getting to know myself on a deeper level, connecting with others on a deeper level and understanding their drives, and designing an environment they wanted to be a part of while leading them towards changing behaviors, attitudes, values, and beliefs.

The self-determination theory suggests that people are motivated to grow and change by three innate and universal psychological needs: autonomy, competence, and connection.

Autonomy: people need to feel in control of their own behaviors and goals and have a sense of being able to take direct action that will result in change.

Competence: when people feel like they have the skills needed for success, they are more likely to take actions that will help them achieve their goals.

Connection: people need to experience a sense of belonging and attachment to other people.

Upon reading those statements, the initial reaction might be "duh." But how often are we taking into consideration these psycho-social and psycho-emotional aspects of human behavior when we think about the type of culture or environment we want to create? Or when it comes to maximizing one's full potential?

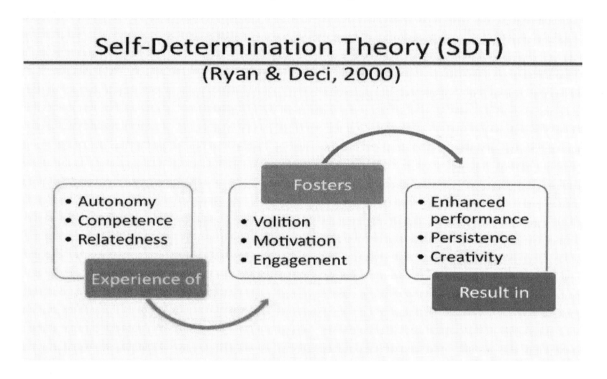

Shepelek, R 2019 https://sites.google.com/site/learnteachtech/home/learning-theory/self-determination

The first step is connection. If we truly want to maximize an athlete's potential, we must set out to win their hearts and minds. This comes from taking the time to get curious and focus on getting to know them on a personal level. My focus has shifted from "What do we need to get accomplished?" to "Who is the person standing in front of me and what is their experience?" When an athlete first steps foot on campus, I meet with them individually and just talk. I'm not explaining my philosophy or what we are going to do that's going to help – I'm asking questions about who they are and I'm listening. Eventually I ask questions about training background…What do you like to do? What do you dislike? What do you feel like helps you the most? These questions, along with others, help drive input and decision making. The most important question I ask is; what is the desirable, yet difficult to reach, future you see for yourself? When it is clear where they want to go and what drives them, every decision and behavior can be tied back to that. My approach is to earn their trust and respect over time by meeting them where they are and building a relationship with them that is strong enough to handle the truth. Truth is powerful – we must be able to live it, tell it, and take it. That only becomes possible if the connection is strong enough. If I don't take the time to get to know my athletes and connect what we are doing to what they care about and where they want to go, how can they ever trust and believe what I'm doing is in their best interest?

Education is key in developing an athlete's competence in the weight room. I do my best to educate them on the process and the "why" behind everything we do. I want them to understand their bodies, how to train, and how to make decisions regarding training when I am not in the room and when they leave after their collegiate career is over. This takes a tremendous amount of work on the front end. I encourage them to ask questions and challenge me. I've learned that true leadership shows an incredible amount of vulnerability. I am no longer afraid to admit I may not have all the answers and no longer feel the need to control every aspect of training. By educating them, involving them in the process, and allowing them to have a say, they become empowered to make decisions and take ownership of their development. It is important to note, however, that while education is key, it must be delivered in a way that caters to emotion and what the athlete truly cares about. Teenage brains are driven by emotion, not logic, and emotion will trump logic every time. Delivering information is only as effective as it can be connected, and it is our responsibility to find ways for our athletes to listen (see previous paragraph on connection).

What I have ultimately tried to develop at the University of South Carolina is a player-led culture and autonomous environment. This does not mean they run the show or are the sole decision makers, it simply means they are given a voice, choices, and empowered to make decisions for themselves and the team. When an athlete has a vote and a voice, the work becomes more meaningful because it was their decision. Many coaches view a successful culture as one where there is compliance or obedience. While compliance may yield short-term results, the growth that occurs is not as significant. I have become less concerned with short-term outcomes and more focused on playing the long game of development. My role has shifted from dictator to facilitator. I serve as a guide to help them navigate training, basketball, and life.

This type of leadership requires an incredible amount of humility and a relentless internal battle with our own ego. Furthermore, it is undoubtedly a continuous, imperfect process. When we can accept that learning and growth are messy and nonlinear, it becomes much easier to adopt this style. Training sessions will not look perfect. It is messy and sometimes it will feel unproductive or ineffective – and that's okay. True growth only occurs by allowing people the space to fail, work through things, and learn from their mistakes without the fear of punishment or consequences.

As mentioned earlier, letting go of control is hard; yet, when we give up some of that control and give ownership and autonomy to the athletes themselves, a funny thing happens. We gain influence. When we have influence, we have the greatest opportunity to impact people and achieve exponential growth. By forming a partnership, we can grow together. Since encountering the crossroads two years ago, the journey has been messy but the results incredibly rewarding. In that span, we have experienced an undisputed number one ranking before our season was cut short due to COVID, and were one-point shy from playing in a national championship game.

The coloring will continue…

Who is Molly Binetti?

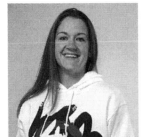

Sports performance coach Molly Binetti brought her athlete-centered coaching philosophy to South Carolina in June 2018, and the Gamecocks immediately responded to her focus on a holistic development of mind, body and spirit.

"Molly's passion for women's basketball was clear right off the bat, and that's the kind of energy we like in our program," South Carolina head coach Dawn Staley said. "Her experience with basketball and other sports gives her great perspective, and her research background shows her commitment to her craft."

Binetti joined the Gamecock staff after four seasons at Louisville working with volleyball, softball and women's tennis. She spent the first three of those seasons as the secondary sports performance coach for women's basketball as well. At Louisville, she focused on power development and applied sport technologies, a trend she continues at South Carolina. Prior to her tenure at Louisville, Binetti served as the sports performance coach for Purdue's women's tennis, men's and women's diving and cheerleading teams (2013-14).

The Eau Claire, Wis., native has her Strength and Conditioning Coach certification from the Collegiate Strength and Conditioning Coaches Association and is listed as a Certified Strength and Conditioning Specialist and a Registered Strength and Conditioning Coach by the National Strength and Conditioning Association. She has contributed to two articles published in the *Journal of Strength and Conditioning Research,* both focused on women's basketball athletes and has attended the USOC High Performance Symposium in Colorado Springs, Colo.

After earning her bachelor's degree in exercise physiology from Marquette in 2012, Binetti completed her master's in kinesiology and exercise science at Minnesota in 2013

Bio from:

https://gamecocksonline.com/sports/womens-basketball/roster/coaches/molly-binetti/935

2

Heavy Strength Training for Sport

The Art and Science of Developing Stronger Athletes

Antonio Squillante

M.S., RSCC, CSCS*D, SENr, CISSN

Traditional strength training for sport makes great use of heavy, compound lifts with weights in excess of 80% of 1RM. To some extent an athlete can control the velocity at which the bar moves during the concentric portion of the movement, although accelerating becomes harder and harder as the weight gets heavier.

Percentage-Based Training and Velocity-Based Training

If the load dictates the number of repetitions an athlete must complete each set, then heavy strength training is referred to as *prescription-based training* or *percentage-based training* (PBT). On average, an athlete is capable of completing 80% to 90% of the maximum number of repetitions possible or RM per set – *for instance, at 80% of 1RM or 8RM only 5-6 repetitions are performed* – before the onset of fatigue can compromise muscle function (11, 23, 33). Sets of *2-4* repetitions are routinely performed with weights ranging between 85% and 95% of 1RM, with more experienced, stronger athletes who might be able to undergo eccentric training with loads in excess of 120% of 1RM. On the other hand, if average vertical bar velocity dictates the number of repetitions an athlete can complete each set, then heavy strength training is referred to as *velocity-based training* (VBT). On average, an athlete is capable of completing only 50% of the maximum number of repetitions possible (RM) – *for instance, at 80% of 1RM or 8RM only 3-4 repetitions are performed with an average vertical bar velocity of 0.5 m·sec^{-1}* – before average vertical bar velocity starts to decline (18, 19, 36). Sets of *3-5* repetitions are routinely performed with weights ranging between 75% and 85% of 1RM, with more experienced, stronger athletes who might be able to complete repetitions at 0.5 m·sec^{-1} with somewhat of a heavier load.

HEAVY STRENGTH TRAINING Load-Repetitions Range			
1RM LOAD	**RM** REPETITIONS	**PBT**	**VBT**
100%	1	--	--
95%	2	1	--
90%	3	2	--
85%	5	3	3
80%	8	4	4
75%	10	6	5
70%	12	10	6

Heavy strength training load-repetition range. *Adapted from*: Squillante, A. (2021). *Power. The Training of Champions*. Ultimate Athlete Concepts. Maximum repetitions are based on: Haff, G. G., & Triplett, N. T. (2015). *Essentials of Strength Training and Conditioning 4th Edition*. Human kinetics.

Heavy VBT – *i.e. basic, compound lifts with weights equal to or greater than 75% of 1RM and average vertical bar velocity of about 0.5-0.7 m·sec^{-1}* – can be considered as a valuable alternative to heavy PBT in strength training for sport. Evidence has shown the benefit of training at higher velocity on muscular strength, sheer power, and rate of force development. A study published by *The Journal of Strength and Conditioning Research* in 2020 has compared VBT to PBT in a group of 16 subjects who underwent 6 weeks of heavy strength training. Eight subjects followed a more traditional PBT program whereas 8 subjects followed what can be considered heavy VBT training. Jump height and muscular strength were measured before and after training. VBT resulted in a greater improvement in lower and upper body strength, on average 18% more than PBT. VBT only resulted in an appreciable increase in jumping height (5%). VBT not only improves muscle function to a greater extent than heavy PBT but it also decreases the total training volume an athlete must undergo. A difference of approximately 10% in load between PBT and VBT, that multiplied repetition after repetition, set after set, corresponds to a significant difference in volume load between the two groups. If the load were to be the same, VBT would count, on average, for only two-thirds to half the number of repetitions of a traditional PBT program (33, 36)

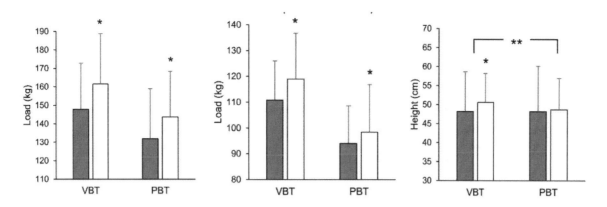

Retrieved from: Dorrell, H. F., Smith, M. F., & Gee, T. I. (2020). Comparison of velocity-based and traditional percentage-based loading methods on maximal strength and power adaptations. The Journal of Strength & Conditioning Research, 34(1), 46-53. From left to right: Back Squat (1), Bench Press, Countermovement Jump

VBT rarely allows the use of loads in excess of 85% of 1RM. This is a necessary compromise to preserve a relatively constant average vertical bar velocity of approximately 0.5 $m{\cdot}sec^{-1}$ (± 10-20%). The load-velocity tradeoff in VBT can be explained by looking at the basic mechanics of muscle contraction and the effect of fatigue on the neuromuscular system. In the early XIX century, the British physiologist, and Nobel Prize in Physiology or Medicine winner, Archibald Vivian Hill (1886-1977) explained in great detail the effect of velocity on the mechanics of muscle contraction (17). As the velocity of muscle contraction increases, force decreases and vice versa. The strength of this basic assumption is such that greater power is generated when neither force nor velocity of muscle contraction is at its peak (14, 21). McBride and colleagues (2011) have done an outstanding job collecting data on ground reaction force, peak vertical bar velocity, and peak power output in a variety of different exercises, each one corresponding to a different regimen of muscle contraction. In the back squat, for instance, for incremental loads up to 90% of 1RM, force peaks at 90% of 1RM whereas vertical bar velocity is greater at lower loads. Peak power output in heavy, compound lifts occur when ground force equals roughly 80% of peak ground reaction force and vertical bar velocity corresponding to 65% of peak vertical bar velocity (26).

FORCE-VELOCITY PROFILE McBride, et al. (2011)			
Load 1RM	Peak Power Output (watt)	Peak Force (kg)	Peak Velocity (m·sec⁻¹)
0%	1005 ± 342	1326 ± 171	1.10 ± 0.25
10%	1123 ± 360	1492 ± 228	1.03 ± 028
20%	1167 ± 426	1558 ± 272	0.98 ± 0.25
30%	1148 ± 329	1683 ± 294	0.87 ± 0.19
40%	1165 ± 411	1802 ± 259	0.80 ± 0.23
50%	1840 ± 405	1956 ± 287	0.73 ± 0.18
60%	1065 ± 218	2060 ± 290	0.62 ± 0.12
70%	1001 ± 406	2180± 317	0.53 ± 0.19
80%	771± 346	2302 ± 288	0.39 ± 0.16
90%	746 ± 333	2447 ± 287	0.35 ± 0.16

Retrieved from: McBride, J. M., Haines, T. L., & Kirby, T. J. (2011). Effect of loading on peak power of the bar, body, and system during power cleans, squats, and jump squats. Journal of Sports Sciences, 29(11), 1215-1221.

In order to increase the amount of force being generated during voluntary muscle contractions, greater effort is required. Greater effort – *i.e. lifting heavier weights and/or lifting the same weight at a higher velocity* – requires a larger number of motor units to be recruited. Fast-twitch motor units contribute to force production during heavy lifting, making it possible to generate explosive muscle contractions. These are fast-glycolytic muscle fibers – *fast-twitch muscle fibers or type II muscle fibers are often referred to as fast glycolytic (FG) fibers* – and despite their ability to generate high levels of force, FG muscle fibers also fatigue very rapidly. As the number of repetitions per set increases, the turnover rate between fast-twitch muscle and slow-twitch muscle fibers increases. As FG muscle fibers get fatigued, a greater number of slow-twitch or slow-oxidative (SO) muscle fibers are recruited. So, muscle fibers have a much lower threshold of activation, yet their ability to generate force is significantly lower than FG muscle fibers. Therefore, as the number of repetitions per set increases, average vertical bar velocity inevitably declines (25, 28).

For a load equal to or greater than 80% of 1RM average vertical bar velocity – *in good approximation, an estimate of the velocity of muscle contraction* – declines with an increase in the number of repetitions being performed. Each set might begin with an average vertical bar velocity of 0.5 m·sec^{-1}. However, the onset of fatigue limits the ability to carry on explosive muscle contractions, and average vertical bar velocity at the end of a set of 3-5 repetitions might drop below 0.4 m·sec^{-1}. By using lighter weights – *on average, anywhere between 70% and 80% of 1RM* – or, simply, by performing fewer and fewer repetitions per set, roughly 50% of the number of repetitions, an athlete could complete the set before muscle failure. Thus, it is possible to prevent fatigue from hindering muscle function. Managing fatigue, in turn, makes it possible to keep average vertical bar velocity at or above 0.5 m·sec^{-1}. Shorter sets, lighter weights, and longer rest periods have a profound effect on average vertical bar velocity (2, 33). A compelling amount of evidence has corroborated the importance of preserving muscle function during training in order to elicit a greater, more profound level of neuromuscular adaptation (10, 14). Studies have also suggested a strong correlation between average power output during heavy strength training and serum testosterone concentration, a factor that plays a major role in driving adaptation (13, 31).

There are, undoubtedly, many benefits of using heavy VBT when striving to improve muscular strength. However, there are important limitations as well. One possible source of limitation, and to some extent a more trivial one, is the limited hypertrophic response to VBT. Muscle growth or muscle hypertrophy heavily relies on an increased rate of protein synthesis which is commonly associated with a greater volume of training (30) . For those athletes who might need to increase lean body mass to be able to generate greater-than-average levels of sheer strength – for a male athlete more than 2-2.2 times bodyweight in the barbell back squat (1RM), for a female athlete more than 1.5-1.8 times bodyweight in the barbell back squat (1RM) – greater muscle mass becomes necessary to improve performance in sport. Strength does, in fact, increase more or less linearly with an increase in muscle cross-sectional area (CSA). However, for the vast majority of athletes, an increase in lean body mass may not be necessary. Excessive muscle mass might, indeed, become counterproductive as it can potentially lower the power-to-weight ratio and negatively affect performance in sports that require high levels of acceleration and/or linear speed. VBT may very well fit the needs of those athletes who do not necessarily require high volumes of training and/or greater-than-average levels of muscular development.

The second source of limitation, and by far, a more important one to consider when it comes to strength training for sport, is the lack of exposure to near-maximal loads during training. Near-maximal loads (>90% 1RM) are necessary to increase muscle-tendon stiffness, the ability of the muscle-tendon complex to store and use elastic energy during explosive, plyometric-like, muscle actions. Both active stiffness – *a function of muscular strength, as greater strength increases the ability to withstand deformation during eccentric overloading* – and passive stiffness – *the inherent resistance to passive deformation of the skeletal muscle tissue due to its viscous-elastic properties* – are of paramount importance in developing stronger, more powerful athletes. Eccentric overload, a prerogative of heavy strength training for sport, increases the content and the size of a protein known as titin, the largest protein ever to be isolated (9, 16). Titin provides integrity to the sarcomere by running from the Z-disc to the M-line while holding together actin and myosin filaments in well-organized, geometrically-sounded structures. By doing so, titin plays a major role in improving both active and passive muscle stiffness. The spring-like properties of this protein allow for a muscle to resist deformation when exposed to eccentric loading (15). Moreover, the Ca^{2+} mediated interaction between titin and actin increases muscle stiffness during dynamic muscle actions (12, 27).

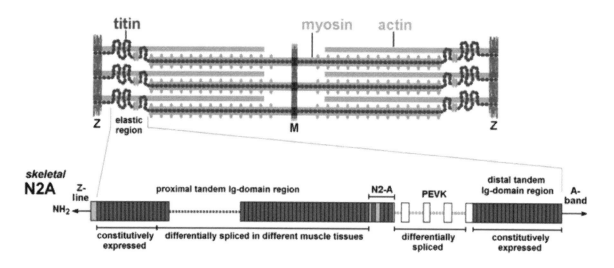

Retrieved from: Neagoe, C., Opitz, C. A., Makarenko, I., & Linke, W. A. (2003). Gigantic variety: expression patterns of titin isoforms in striated muscles and consequences for myofibrillar passive stiffness. Journal of Muscle Research & Cell Motility, 24(2), 175-189.

Greater titin content in skeletal muscle not only improves muscle function by increasing strength, power, and rate of force development, but also prevents muscles from undergoing severe damage during eccentric overloading, a condition that is often associated with the most common mechanism of injury in sport. Eccentric overloading not only increases the titin content in skeletal muscle fibers but also increases the content of $N_2A(S)$ titin-isoforms, which further contributes to increase muscle stiffness (29, 35). An increase in titin content often occurs with a simultaneous increase in size and strength of the extracellular matrix (ECM), the serial elastic element surrounding the layers of muscle tissue often referred to as epimysium, perimysium, and endomysium (7, 22). Despite the many benefits associated with the use of near-maximal load, and arguably so, supramaximal loads within the context of eccentric strength training (120-140% 1RM), heavy, traditional PBT might have important limitations as well. Training at lower velocity can, indeed, alter the mechanics of muscle contraction resulting in a less efficient and effective rate of force development (RDF) during ballistic, explosive movements. Training at greater velocity is, in fact, a necessity when the goal is to improve muscle function. Traditional PBT with near-maximal load might provide an ideal situation to improve absolute strength, but it fails to provide athletes with the necessary level of physiological adaptation needed to improve speed, power, and agility.

In a study published by *The Journal of Strength and Conditioning Research* in 2002, McBride and colleagues compared 8 weeks of strength training with heavy squat jumps at 80% of 1RM with 8 weeks of strength training with lighter squat jumps at 30% of 1RM. Speed, power, and agility were measured before and after training, and electromyographic (EMG) activity was recorded for each subject during a jump squat at 30%, 55%, or 80% of 1RM. Training with heavier loads improved peak force and peak power outputs during heavier jump squats (>55% 1RM) but it showed no correlation with any other key performance variable. Training with lighter weights, on the other hand, improved peak force and peak power outputs during the jump squat with lighter loads (<55% 1RM), with more remarkable improvement in speed, power, and agility. The change in EMG activity explains these results. Previous studies have shown how training at a higher velocity results in greater EMG activity than training with heavier weights, leading to a greater, more meaningful change in muscle function along the entire force-velocity curve (3, 24).

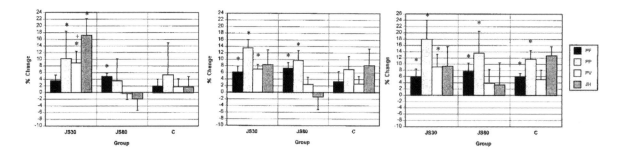

Retrieved from: McBride, J. M., Triplett-McBride, T., Davie, A., & Newton, R. U. (2002). The effect of heavy-vs. light-load jump squats on the development of strength, power, and speed. The Journal of Strength & Conditioning Research, 16(1), 75-82.

Compensatory Acceleration Training

The use of *compensatory acceleration training* (CAT), also known as *intended maximal concentric acceleration* (IMCA) training, might preserve the benefit of using near-maximal loads while avoiding the detrimental effects of heavy lifting on neuromuscular performance. CAT utilizes heavy weights (>80% of 1RM) to develop muscular strength. The term compensatory is used to describe the assumption behind the use of IMCA training. EMG activity during heavy lifting varies widely throughout the entire range of motion. The results of a study published in 2017 by the scientific journal *Applied Bionics and Biomechanics* have helped to map the average profile of neuromuscular activation in traditional, heavy compound lifts such as squats, pulls, and presses. For this particular study, the EMG profile of the main musculature of the lower extremity was recorded during a barbell back squat for incremental loads of 80%, 90%, and 100% of 1RM. Similar considerations apply to different compound, core lifts. EMG activity has been shown to vary quite drastically throughout the concentric portion of the movement. Motor unit recruitment in the knee extensor musculature – *vastus medialis, vastus lateralis, and rectus femoris*– peaks at the transition between eccentric and concentric muscle action whereas the knee flexors and hip extensor muscle – *semimembranosus, bicep femoris, and gluteus maximus* – are co-activated to create the necessary degree of joint stability under a condition of greater load. EMG activity sharply declines as the concentric muscle actions take place (37). This unique pattern of muscle activation is attributable to the inherent mechanical features of the vast majority of compound, core lifts with the exception of weightlifting.

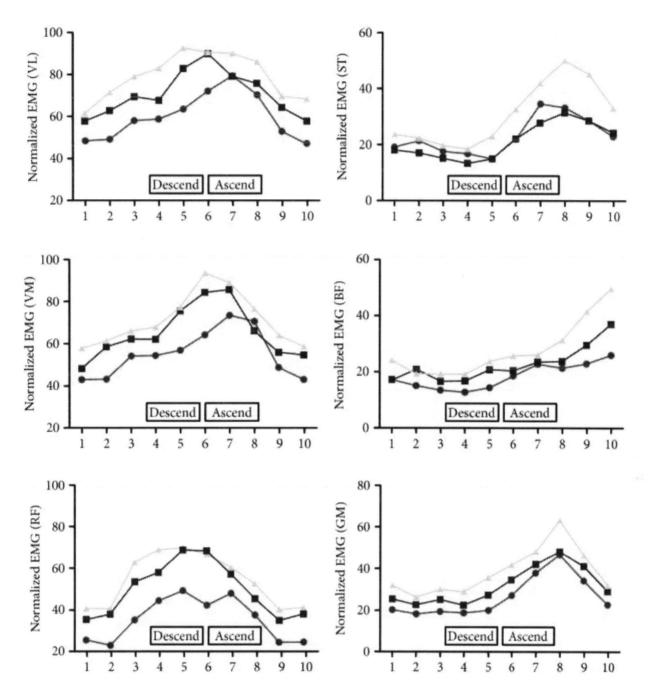

Retrieved from: Yavuz, H. U., & Erdag, D. (2017). Kinematic and electromyographic activity changes during back squat with submaximal and maximal loading. Applied bionics and biomechanics, 2017. Muscle recruitment in a maximal (100% 1RM ▲) and submaximal (80% 1RM ▲ and 90% 1RM ▲) barbell back squat measured via electromyography (EMG). In order: rectus femoris (RF), vastus medialis (VM), vastus lateralis (VL), erector spinae (ES), gluteus maximus (GM), biceps femoris (BF), and semitendinosus (ST).

Despite a relatively straight bar path, core lifts represent quite a complex mechanical system. An athlete's center of mass (CM) can be placed with good approximation at the level of L5-S1. Its perpendicular distance from the line of application of the force – *i.e. moment arm* – increases during the eccentric portion of the movement and decreases during the concentric portion of the lift. The amount of external resistance does not change throughout the entire range of motion, and for this very reason compound core lifts can be considered as true isotonic exercises. However, the sheer load placed upon the neuromuscular system does change during the concentric portion of the movement as the moment arm changes, affecting the degree to which motor units are recruited. A longer moment arm corresponds to a situation of mechanical disadvantage. Hence, the neuromuscular system must generate an increased amount of torque – *torque (or moment) = F·d with d=perpendicular distance from the line of application of the force to the center of rotation of the join* – to overcome inertia. Greater torque can be generated if a larger number of motor units are recruited (intramuscular coordination) or a larger number of muscle groups participate together resulting in greater net force to be applied against the ground (intramuscular coordination). On the other hand, a shorter moment arm corresponds to a situation of mechanical advantage, and the neuromuscular system must no longer generate an increased amount of torque to overcome inertia. Therefore, motor unit recruitment tends to decrease.

Greater adaptation to resistance training has been shown to occur when the combination between the force generated and the velocity of muscle contraction elicits a greater level of neuromuscular activation (3, 6, 20). Force increases as the load on the bar increases. However, the change in moment arm that occurs during the concentric portion of the movement might alter the force-velocity profile of a given muscle/muscle group, and only a greater voluntary effort to accelerate the bar can compensate for the increase in mechanical advantage while preserving a greater rate of motor unit recruitment and synchronization. Hence, the term *compensatory* being used to describe this alternative approach to traditional, heavy PBT. Although CAT does strive to increase acceleration, nearing the completion of the set the average vertical bar velocity might drop below 0.5 m·sec^{-1}. Therefore, CAT must not be confused with VBT. A study published by *The Journal of Strength and Conditioning Research in* 1999 has shown the benefit of training with greater acceleration – CAT – when compared to traditional strength training for sport. A group of 40 collegiate NCAA Division 1AA American football players underwent 14 weeks of upper body strength training. After three weeks of general physical preparedness, one group performed heavy sets of 3-5 repetitions at or above 80% of 1RM, up to 95% of 1RM, with 2 minutes of rest between sets. The experimental group performed each set striving for the greatest acceleration possible at each repetition. Average vertical bar velocity declined as the load progressively increased varying quite largely from lighter sets – 0.6 m·sec^{-1} at 75% of 1RM – to heavier sets – 0.4 m·sec^{-1} at 90% of 1RM – with a decline of approximately 40-60% from the first repetition to the last repetition of each set. The control group carried on with traditional strength training. Average vertical bar velocity in the control group varied between 0.3 m·sec^{-1} and 0.5 m·sec^{-1}, with a similar rate of decline from the first repetition to the last repetition of each set. Hence, vertical bar velocity, per se, did not vary in an appreciable manner between groups.

COMPENSATORY ACCELERATION TRAINING Table 1 - Jones, et al (1999)				
Test	**Seated Medicine Ball Throw** Explosive Strength		**Bench Press 1RM** Absolute Strength	
Results	Traditional	CAT	Traditional	CAT
Pre	7.9 ± 0.5	7.3 ± 0.4	130.0 ± 18.2	114.7 ± 17.2
Post	8.1 ± 0.6	8.0 ± 0.5	135.0 ± 19.0	125.5 ± 15.5
Change	+0.2	+0.7	+5.0	+9.8
% Change	+2.8	+9.4	+3.8	+8.6

Adapted from: Jones, K., Hunter, G., FLEISIG, G., Escamilla, R., & Lemak, L. (1999). The effects of compensatory acceleration on upper-body strength and power in collegiate football players. The Journal of Strength & Conditioning Research, 13(2), 99-105.

The results of a series of tests performed at the end of the training intervention revealed quite a significant difference in training adaptation between the two groups. Each subject was tested for upper body strength (bench press 1RM) and power (seated medicine ball throw). Moreover, a plyometric push-up was used to measure average power, amortization time, and peak force during ballistic-like, explosive muscle actions. The experimental group showed a much more significant change in upper body strength (+8.6% compared to +3.8%) and power (+9.4% compared to +2.8%) compared to the control group. Training with intended maximal concentric acceleration not only improved strength in the upper extremities but also improved efficiency in the stretch-shortening cycle. The length of the amortization phase during the stretch-shortening cycle decreased (-0.046 compared to -0.022 milliseconds) and peak power output increased (+365 W compared to +108 W) to a greater extent in the experimental group although peak force did not improve as much (+70 N compared to +95 N), suggesting how a greater rate of force development must have been responsible for a more powerful concentric muscle action. Results from this study confirm, or at the very least suggest, that heavy strength training might indeed improve power just as much, if not more, than explosive strength training, when athletes make a conscious effort to maximally accelerate the weight during the concentric portion of the movement (5, 38).

Accommodative Resistance Training

It is possible to use additional resistance in the form of elastic bands and chains to create a variable amount of load throughout the concentric portion of basic, compound lifts such as squats, pulls, and presses. This method is known as *accommodative resistance training* (ART). As the chains unfold from the ground up and/or elastic bands are stretched during the concentric portion of the lift, the amount of the external load increases while mechanical disadvantage decreases, compensating for the lack of internal load. It is possible to modulate the relative contribution of the true inertial mass – *i.e. the weight on the barbell* – and the additional resistance in the form of chains and bands. The net load varies, on average, from 40% to 80% of 1RM with roughly 20-30% of additional resistance coming from chains and bands. The relative percentage of inertial resistance must be such that at the so-called sticking point, the point at which the moment arm is the longest creating a situation of mechanical disadvantage, the weight on the bar does not exceed 70-80% of 1RM for the development of absolute strength or 30-40% of 1RM for the development of explosive strength. Elastic bands and chains can then provide an additional amount of resistance: up to 10-20% for heavy strength training, for a total load on the bar equal to or greater than 90% of 1RM, and up to 20-30% for explosive strength training, for a total load on the bar equal to or greater than 60% of 1RM (1, 4, 34). As the load increases, the pattern of motor unit recruitment and synchronization changes quite drastically. On one hand, when training to improve muscular strength it is possible to maximize the amount of additional load coming from bands and chains to match an athlete's 1RM, as long as the number of repetitions performed changes accordingly. On the other hand, when training to improve power and rate of force development it is of paramount importance to limit the additional load coming from bands and chains to match the optimal load to maximize peak power output in basic, compound lifts which corresponds, roughly, to 60-70% of 1RM.

Recent studies have compared the effect of accommodative resistance training on muscle strength to more traditional heavy strength training and explosive strength training exercises. A study published by *The Journal of Strength and Conditioning Research* in 2009 has compared explosive strength training with accommodative resistance to traditional heavy strength training and explosive ballistic strength training. 48 NCAA Division I athletes underwent 12 weeks of lower body strength training. Exercises were kept similar between groups, with the only exception of the barbell back squat: one group performed heavy sets with an average vertical bar velocity of 0.2-0.4m·sec^{-1} (Slow), one group performed lighter sets with an average vertical bar velocity of 0.6-0.8 m·sec^{-1} (Fast), and a third group performed lighter sets with the addition of elastic bands and similar vertical bar velocity of 0.6-0.8 m·sec^{-1} (FACC). Subjects were tested before and after the 12-week intervention measuring a change in lower body strength (barbell back squat 1RM) and power (countermovement vertical jump).

POWER Rhea, et al (2009)			
Group	**Pre-Test (W)**	**Post-Test (W)**	**Change**
Slow	1151 ± 205.62	1208.31 ± 24.78	4.8%
Fast	1124.75 ± 174.25	1264.25 ± 192.37	11%
FACC	1146.38 ± 226.41	1387.19 ± 221.65	17.8%

MUSCULAR STRENGTH Rhea, et al (2009)			
Group	**Pre-Test (1RM)**	**Post-Test (1RM)**	**Change**
Slow	122.31± 39.04	131.94 ± 3.43	9.59%
Fast	115.94 ± 36.07	119.18 ± 35.56	3.2%
FACC	116.00 ± 31.43	125.81 ± 30.69	9.44%

Adapted from: Rhea, M. R., Kenn, J. G., & Dermody, B. M. (2009). Alterations in speed of squat movement and the use of accommodated resistance among college athletes training for power. The Journal of Strength & Conditioning Research, 23(9), 2645-2650.

Performance in the barbell back squat improved to a similar extent in both slow and FACC groups, whereas the change was not as appreciable in the fast group. Peak power output, on the other hand, more noticeably improved in the FACC group, confirming how the use of accommodating resistance might be a valuable alternative to more traditional explosive strength training. ART does, indeed, develop strength and power to a larger extent than traditional, ballistic-like explosive lifts. However, its effect of absolute strength when compared to traditional, heavy strength training is trivial. These findings have been corroborated by a series of meta-analyses confirming no additional benefit in using chains and bands compared to traditional, heavy strength training (8, 32). The advantage of accommodating resistance training seems to be limited to explosive strength training for sport with the contingency of applying the appropriate amount of load (30-60% of 1RM) and preserving the optimal average vertical bar velocity (0.7-0.8 m·sec[-1]) in the attempt to yield greater mechanical power output. Despite the similarities between CAT and VBT, there are some important differences in the way these training modalities are used to develop strength and power in sport.

Maximal Intended Velocity

A study published by the scientific journal *Applied Sports Sciences* in 2014 has shown the benefit of training with maximal intended velocity. For this study, 6 weeks of strength training were performed using progressive resistance training with loads starting at 60% of 1RM (3 sets of 6-8 repetitions) up to 80% of 1RM (3 sets of 2-3 repetitions). Each subject was instructed to strive for the greatest possible vertical bar velocity during the concentric portion of the movement although vertical bar velocity dropped quite significantly during each working set, falling below 0.5 $m \cdot sec^{-1}$. Training with maximal intended velocity not only resulted in a significant increase in absolute strength (1RM) but also resulted in greater vertical bar velocity at different loads, both submaximal loads (<50% 1RM) and near-maximal loads (>80% 1RM), suggesting a significant increase in mechanical power (25, 28).

MAXIMUM INTENDED VELOCITY TRAINING González-Badillo et al (2014)						
Variable	Pre	Post	Δ (%)	Pre	Post	Δ (%)
Strength 1RM	75.8 ± 17.9	88.2 ± 15.1	18.2 ± 11.9	73.9 ± 9.7	80.8 ± 11.2	9.7 ± 7.9
MPV_{avg} $m \cdot s^{-1}$	0.76 ± 0.09	0.91 ± 0.08	20.8 ± 9.6	0.75 ± 0.07	0.83 ± 0.09	10.0 ± 7.2
MPV_{avg} > 0.8 $m \cdot s^{-1}$	1.03 ± 0.11	1.15 ± 0.10	11.5 ± 6.5	1.03 ± 0.08	1.08 ± 0.12	4.5 ± 6.1
MPV_{avg} < 0.8 $m \cdot s^{-1}$	0.55 ± 0.06	0.74 ± 0.06	36.2 ± 20.0	0.55 ± 0.05	0.64 ± 0.08	17.3 ± 11.3

Adapted from: González-Badillo, J. J., Rodríguez-Rosell, D., Sánchez-Medina, L., Gorostiaga, E. M., & Pareja-Blanco, F. (2014). Maximal intended velocity training induces greater gains in bench press performance than deliberately slower half-velocity training. European Journal of Sport Science, 14(8), 772-781.

Conclusion

When training to improve absolute strength, a lower vertical bar velocity in exchange for greater acceleration against heavier loads can be as productive as training at higher velocity with lighter loads. The effect of movement velocity during progressive resistance training on muscle function and neuromuscular performance has been well documented over the last few decades. Werner Günthör, a three-time World Champion in the shotput and medalist at the 1988 Summer Olympics, trained with maximal intended velocity during the 1991-1992 season. In 6 weeks, Günthör's peak power output in the barbell back squat went from 1,473 W for a load corresponding to 180 kg to 1,737 W for a load corresponding to 220 kg. Günthör not only was capable of generating more power, but he was indeed capable of generating more power against heavier and heavier loads, the true ultimate goal of strength training for sport. Limitations in the so-called PBT approach to strength training compared to VBT are inherent to the degree of effort an athlete is willing to put in training. Controlling for velocity and adjusting loads accordingly to match the ability of an athlete to overcome inertia with greater acceleration is the key to keep an athlete honest day in and day out, optimizing training to improve performance in sport.

REFERENCES

1. Anderson CE, Sforzo GA, and Sigg JA. The effects of combining elastic and free weight resistance on strength and power in athletes. *The Journal of Strength & Conditioning Research* 22: 567-574, 2008.

2. Arazi H, Khanmohammadi A, Asadi A, and Haff GG. The effect of resistance training set configuration on strength, power, and hormonal adaptation in female volleyball players. *Applied physiology, nutrition, and metabolism* 43: 154-164, 2018.

3. Behm D and Sale D. Velocity specificity of resistance training. *Sports medicine* 15: 374-388, 1993.

4. Bellar DM, Muller MD, Barkley JE, Kim C-H, Ida K, Ryan EJ, Bliss MV, and Glickman EL. The effects of combined elastic-and free-weight tension vs. free-weight tension on one-repetition maximum strength in the bench press. *The Journal of Strength & Conditioning Research* 25: 459-463, 2011.

5. Bosco C, Belli A, Astrua M, Tihanyi J, Pozzo R, Kellis S, Tsarpela O, Foti C, Manno R, and Tranquilli C. A dynamometer for evaluation of dynamic muscle work. *European journal of applied physiology and occupational physiology* 70: 379-386, 1995.

6. Bosco C, Ito A, Komi P, Luhtanen P, Rahkila P, Rusko H, and Viitasalo J. Neuromuscular function and mechanical efficiency of human leg extensor muscles during jumping exercises. *Acta physiologica scandinavica* 114: 543-550, 1982.

7. Csapo R, Gumpenberger M, and Wessner B. Skeletal muscle extracellular matrix–what do we know about its composition, regulation, and physiological roles? A narrative review. *Frontiers in physiology* 11: 253, 2020.

8. de Oliveira PA, Blasczyk JC, Junior GS, Lagoa KF, Soares M, de Oliveira RJ, Gutierres Filho PJB, Carregaro RL, and Martins WR. Effects of elastic resistance exercise on muscle strength and functional performance in healthy adults: a systematic review and meta-analysis. *Journal of physical activity and health* 14: 317-327, 2017.

9. Douglas J, Pearson S, Ross A, and McGuigan M. Eccentric exercise: physiological characteristics and acute responses. *Sports Medicine* 47: 663-675, 2017.

10. Duchateau J and Hainaut K. Mechanisms of muscle and motor unit adaptation to explosive power training. *Strength and power in sport*: 315, 2003.

11. Duffey MJ and Challis JH. Fatigue effects on bar kinematics during the bench press. *Journal of Strength and Conditioning Research* 21: 556, 2007.

12. Dutta S, Tsiros C, Sundar SL, Athar H, Moore J, Nelson B, Gage MJ, and Nishikawa K. Calcium increases titin N2A binding to F-actin and regulated thin filaments. *Scientific reports* 8: 1-11, 2018.

13. Fry A and Lohnes C. Acute testosterone and cortisol responses to high power resistance exercise. *Human physiology* 36: 457-461, 2010.

14. Haff GG and Nimphius S. Training principles for power. *Strength & Conditioning Journal* 34: 2-12, 2012.

15. Herzog W, Schappacher G, DuVall M, Leonard TR, and Herzog JA. Residual force enhancement following eccentric contractions: a new mechanism involving titin. *Physiology* 31: 300-312, 2016.

16. Hessel AL, Lindstedt SL, and Nishikawa KC. Physiological mechanisms of eccentric contraction and its applications: a role for the giant titin protein. *Frontiers in physiology* 8: 70, 2017.

17. Hill AV. The mechanics of active muscle. *Proceedings of the Royal Society of London Series B-Biological Sciences* 141: 104-117, 1953.

18. Hughes LJ, Banyard HG, Dempsey AR, Peiffer JJ, and Scott BR. Using load-velocity relationships to quantify training-induced fatigue. *The Journal of Strength & Conditioning Research* 33: 762-773, 2019.

19. Jovanović M and Flanagan EP. Researched applications of velocity based strength training. *J Aust Strength Cond* 22: 58-69, 2014.

20. Kanehisa H and Miyashita M. Specificity of velocity in strength training. *European journal of applied physiology and occupational physiology* 52: 104-106, 1983.

21. Kawamori N and Haff GG. The optimal training load for the development of muscular power. *The Journal of Strength & Conditioning Research* 18: 675-684, 2004.

22. Kjaer M. Role of extracellular matrix in adaptation of tendon and skeletal muscle to mechanical loading. *Physiological reviews* 84: 649-698, 2004.

23. Lawton TW, Cronin JB, and Lindsell RP. Effect of interrepetition rest intervals on weight training repetition power output. *Journal of Strength and Conditioning Research* 20: 172, 2006.

24. Lesmes GR, Costill DL, Coyle EF, and Fink WJ. Muscle strength and power changes during maximal isokinetic training. *Med Sci Sports* 10: 266-269, 1978.

25. Martínez-Cava A, Morán-Navarro R, Sánchez-Medina L, González-Badillo JJ, and Pallarés JG. Velocity-and power-load relationships in the half, parallel and full back squat. *Journal of Sports Sciences* 37: 1088-1096, 2019.

26. McBride JM, Haines TL, and Kirby TJ. Effect of loading on peak power of the bar, body, and system during power cleans, squats, and jump squats. *Journal of sports sciences* 29: 1215-1221, 2011.

27. Nishikawa KC, Monroy JA, Uyeno TE, Yeo SH, Pai DK, and Lindstedt SL. Is titin a 'winding filament'? A new twist on muscle contraction. *Proceedings of the royal society B: Biological sciences* 279: 981-990, 2012.

28. Sánchez-Medina L, Pallarés JG, Pérez CE, Morán-Navarro R, and González-Badillo JJ. Estimation of relative load from bar velocity in the full back squat exercise. *Sports Medicine International Open* 1: E80, 2017.

29. Savarese M, Jonson PH, Huovinen S, Paulin L, Auvinen P, Udd B, and Hackman P. The complexity of titin splicing pattern in human adult skeletal muscles. *Skeletal muscle* 8: 1-9, 2018.

30. Schoenfeld BJ, Contreras B, Krieger J, Grgic J, Delcastillo K, Belliard R, and Alto A. Resistance training volume enhances muscle hypertrophy but not strength in trained men. *Medicine and science in sports and exercise* 51: 94, 2019.

31. Smilios I, Tsoukos P, Zafeiridis A, Spassis A, and Tokmakidis SP. Hormonal responses after resistance exercise performed with maximum and submaximum movement velocities. *Applied Physiology, Nutrition, and Metabolism* 39: 351-357, 2014.

32. Soria-Gila MA, Chirosa IJ, Bautista IJ, Baena S, and Chirosa LJ. Effects of variable resistance training on maximal strength: a meta-analysis. *The Journal of Strength & Conditioning Research* 29: 3260-3270, 2015.

33. Tufano JJ, Conlon J, Nimphius S, Brown LE, Seitz L, Williamson B, and Haff GG. Cluster sets maintain velocity and power during high-volume back squats. *Int J Sports Physiol Perform* 11: 885-892, 2016.

34. Wallace BJ, Winchester JB, and McGuigan MR. Effects of elastic bands on force and power characteristics during the back squat exercise. *The Journal of Strength & Conditioning Research* 20: 268-272, 2006.

35. Wang K, McCarter R, Wright J, Beverly J, and Ramirez-Mitchell R. Regulation of skeletal muscle stiffness and elasticity by titin isoforms: a test of the segmental extension model of resting tension. *Proceedings of the National Academy of Sciences* 88: 7101-7105, 1991.

36. Weakley J, Mann B, Banyard H, McLaren S, Scott T, and Garcia-Ramos A. Velocity-based training: From theory to application. *Strength Cond J*: 1-19, 2020.

37. Yavuz HU and Erdag D. Kinematic and electromyographic activity changes during back squat with submaximal and maximal loading. *Applied bionics and biomechanics* 2017, 2017.

38. Young WB and Bilby GE. The effect of voluntary effort to influence speed of contraction on strength, muscular power, and hypertrophy development. *The Journal of Strength & Conditioning Research* 7: 172-178, 1993.

Who is Antonio Squillante?

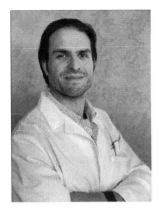

Born and raised in Padova (Italy), Antonio Squillante is a Registered Certified Strength and Conditioning Coach (NSCA RSCC CSCS*D). He graduated Summa Cum Laude with a Bachelor's Degree in Physical Education from the Universita' San Raffaele (Rome, Italy). Antonio earned a Master of Science in Sports Performance and Orthopedic Rehab from A.T. Still University (Mesa, Arizona). With more than a decade of experience working with high school and collegiate athletes competing at national and international level Antonio is considered one of the foremost experts in the field of strength training for sport. His first book "Strength Training for Sport. From Science to Practice" published in 2020 has sold thousands of copies. Antonio is the author of "Power. The Training of Champions" published by Ultimate Athlete Concepts.

3

Beware of Averages

Profiling the Sport and Athlete in Team-Sports for Success

Keir Wenham-Flatt

If we sampled the entire human population, we could be tricked into thinking that an average, normal human being has one breast and one testicle. While averages can sometimes be useful, they can also fool us into poor models of thinking and decision making. A parallel can be drawn into sporting averages...

If we look at the typical distances covered in the NFL, we see players only cover around 1.25 miles over the average 3 hours it takes to play a game, the mean speed achieved is 6/1000ths of a mile per hour. Even if we only account for the 11 minutes of ball in play activity, the mean speed is still around 6.8 mph. Not walking by any means but most healthy adults can jog 1.25 miles at this pace and not be exhausted.

So why do football players get fatigued? Why do we even need to condition for the sport of football? Clearly the problem is not an ability to meet the average demands of the game, but the high intensity demands of the game. To steal from my colleague Mladen Jovanovic, the goal of conditioning for field-based sports like football is:

> "Perform high intensity sporting skills with the greatest possible intensity, frequency, and sustainability possible."

To state the obvious, the high intensity sporting skills that punctuate the game are those which have the greatest impact on the outcome. If two competing athletes are equal in psychological, tactical, and technical preparation (they won't be), the athlete who executes his or her skill with more intensity than their opponent, more often, for longer, wins.

Sport is not about who can work sub-maximally the longest, or who feels freshest in the low intensity activity that intersperses high intensity bursts. In the former, you can just get embarrassed for longer before giving up, and in the latter, you'll arrive earlier to get embarrassed. This is not to say that being able to tolerate a certain level of volume and intensity of work between key contests is not necessary, but when the average demands of the game are akin to the Race for Life, this is clearly not a factor predisposing to success.

Like all aspects of training, it isn't until we've precisely defined what the desired end state looks like before we can reverse engineer a path to navigate athletes from where they are now to where we want them to be with training interventions. Using the broad categories of the "bios" of sport popularised by Verkhoshanky, we can create a profile of the sport and those athletes who are most predisposed to success.

Biodynamics

In the stopwatch sports that the Soviet system was devised to serve, understanding biodynamics is an easy task. It tends to be the sport itself. If you're a shot putter, get really good at the shot. If you're a sprinter, be a master of running. If you're a weightlifter, you need to be an expert of the snatch and clean and jerk.

In the field-based sports, this is a much harder question to ask. Because the demands of field-based sports are inherently more unpredictable, athletes are required to be much more well-rounded. It is conceivable that all football athletes need some basic level of ability in all football skills: catching, throwing, blocking, tackling, hand fighting, sprinting, jumping and cutting. Nonetheless, it is a fact that elite football players tend to make their money being OK at a bunch of stuff, very good at a few things, and truly world class at one or two things. Ask yourself the following questions:

- What do I/they do that is most fatiguing?

- What do I/they do most frequently or better than anyone else on the field?

- What do I/they do that most significantly impacts the outcome of the game?

The answer to these questions are the biodynamic goals you need to work backwards from. Here are my answers, yours may vary:

Offensive line	Lateral movement, blocking
Defensive line	Pass rushing, tackling
Linebackers	Acceleration, tackling
Running backs	Acceleration, cutting
Tight ends	Acceleration, blocking
Safeties	Acceleration, tackling
Cornerbacks	Sprinting, jumping
Wide receivers	Sprinting, jumping
Slot receivers	Sprinting, cutting
Kickers	It's in the name
Quarterbacks	Cutting, throwing

Once we've outlined the primary skills for each position, we can go a level deeper in precisely defining the biomechanical characteristics using another of Verkhoshansky's works- the criteria of dynamic correspondence:

- Muscles used

- Magnitude and direction of force

- Range of motion and peak amplitude of force

- Regime of muscular work

- Sensory information

- Contact time

- Angular velocity

This exercise is useful for establishing hierarchies of more specific or general training exercises used in training to enhance speed of movement in key sporting movements, which is the ultimate goal of all physical preparation. The more criteria a training exercise shares with the sporting skill, the more specific it can be considered and vice versa.

Bio-motor Qualities

Bio-motor qualities describe the categories we use to describe force production potential in a variety of contexts. These can be more general in nature, running the gamut from eccentric strength at one end of the force velocity spectrum to maximal speed at the very opposite end. We can also dig a level deeper and express these qualities per unit of time to arrive at variables like power, rate of force development, and total impulse.

Again, answering the question of which bio-motor qualities to prioritize and which to ignore in the stopwatch sports is an easy exercise. Simply correlate performance in the sport with performance/measurement in that quality. The stronger the correlation, the more predictive ability it has, the more it should be prized for that sport and vice versa. However, in field-based sports like football, the unpredictable and chaotic environment means that all positions need all force production qualities to one degree or another. Nonetheless it is a fair assertion that some qualities will be needed in greater quantities than others.

This can be done two ways: by consulting the list above and the dynamic correspondence to which qualities will be most taxed for a given movement, and by profiling elite athletes in a variety of valid and reliable assessments (which extends beyond the scope of this piece). If you go through this mental exercise you may conclude, as I have, that the closer to the snap a player lines up, the more maximal eccentric, isometric, and concentric strength the athlete needs. As a player lines up further from the snap, the more maximal speed and explosive strength is valued. Players in the box tend to lie between these two extremes. This is confirmed by NFL combine data in which linemen are consistently the strongest, corners and receivers are consistently the fastest, and mid skills are good at both but not excellent at either.

Bioenergetics

Perhaps the most challenging category to evaluate sport demands is bioenergetics. This is because all three energy systems are always "on" and contributing to activity, with the relative contribution of each varying according to the demands of activity. Namely the intensity and duration of work, the work: rest distribution, and the total volume of activity. All of which are subject to tactical-technical strategy, opposition, refereeing etc.

The interactive and interdependent nature of the energy systems means that, as with bio-motor qualities, it is impossible to directly measure and thus define the bio-energetic demands of the sport. In consideration of these difficulties, there are two potential solutions. First is to rely on a battery of highly controlled lab or field-based protocols which allow for isolation and precise measurement of a particular system. A second option is to investigate the time-motion demands of football and try to define what the typical and worst-case pattern of activity looks like.

There is value to both. Diagnostic testing or testing the systems in isolation may be useful for identifying the weak link in the metabolic chain and implementing targeted training interventions, but sustaining high outputs within the context of the game should always be the yardstick by which a conditioning programme is evaluated. It doesn't matter how good your score on the 30:15 or 300yd shuttle test is if you crumble in the game. Conversely, it doesn't matter how poor your score is if you are still able to sustain high outputs longer than your opponent.

Whereas traditional exercise physiology testing is well understood and taught in college and professional education, only a tiny minority of coaches have attempted to define or understand the time motion demands of football, so let's focus on this:

The Time-Motion Demands of American Football

Remarkably only two relevant papers exist on the subject of time-motion demands of football that I am aware of. Though a wealth of research exists regarding the strength characteristics of the athletes, detailed analyses of the pattern of game activity in American Football are lacking.

The relevant studies by Iosia & Bishop, and Rhea, Hunter & Hunter investigated the time motion demands of FBS college football, and NFL, college, and high school football respectively. The findings of these studies can be summarized as follows:

Table 1

Iosia & Bishop (2008)				
Offence style	Time per play (s)	Time between plays without stoppage (s)	Time between plays with stoppage (s)	Rest between drives (mins)
Run	4.86±1.41	35.06±6.03	46.93±37±49	10:53±3:20
Pass	5.6±1.71	38.08±5.85	45.93±24.58	12:15±5:13
Balanced	5.44±1.81	35.21±7.71	47.85±39.10	11:39±4:37

Table 2

Rhea, Hunter & Hunter (2006)			
Play duration (s)			
Play type	**High School**	**College**	**NFL**
Run	5.60±2.04	5.13±1.45	5.16±1.48
Pass	5.68±2.21	5.96±1.62	5.87±1.54
Punt	8.66±2.28	9.82±2.11	8.91±1.96
Kick-off	8.24±4.62	10.39±2.54	11.21±4.50
Play level	**Plays per series**	**Time between plays- no stoppage (s)**	**Time between plays- stoppage (s)**
High school	6.66±3.28	31.49±8.78	81.75±35.81
College	6.26±2.74	33.98±4.19	90.66±47.24
NFL	7.91±3.91	35.24±6.47	112.59±70.48

The mean rest between plays was averaged out over both studies at 34.84s for no stoppages, and 70.95s with stoppages. The Iosia & Bishop study provides no data on mean plays per drive. However, the average plays per drive for high school, college, and NFL per Rhea, Hunter & Hunter was 6.94 plays, with the averaged time between series calculated to be 11 minutes, 29 seconds.

With the omission of kick-off and punt plays, which typically utilise specialist personnel and occur with much lower frequency than standard plays, mean play duration for all levels and all types of play averaged out across both studies to be 5.47s.

Neither study detailed the total number of plays per game, but a quick google search reveals that the average NFL game hovers between 130 and 160 plays total. Assuming an equal split between offense and defense, and a 7 plays per drive average, this equates to anywhere from 9 to 11 drives per game. The real figure is likely to be a little lower when special teams and player rotation is accounted for. Speaking from my own experience of FCS football, a player workload of 60 snaps (about 9 drives) would be considered very high, with most players falling below this number.

Combining the above papers, we can therefore reasonably state that the game of football is approximately 5s of work, 35s of rest, for an average of 7 plays, followed by a substantial rest of 10 minutes or more, repeated for a total of 9 to 11 drives. Based on existing knowledge of exercise physiology and available testing data of top-level players, the game of football is highly alactic-aerobic in nature; the former due to the limited duration and number of plays per drive which reduces reliance on glycolytic energy production, and the latter due to strong correlation of the aerobic system to preserving power output in repeated bouts.

Some Key Considerations

This may look relatively simple on the surface. Train key skills, train the physical abilities that best predict success, train like the game, collect the trophy. Unfortunately, there are a number of conflicting factors we need to keep in our minds, and there is no right answer. In each case it is neither one nor the other, but both. Your ability as a coach to strike the balance between the two, and exercise judgement about when the pendulum should swing from one to the other will have powerful ramifications for the success of your programme.

Typical Case vs. Worst Case

The typical critique from football coaches is that "But we aren't training for the average scenario. We're training for the worst-case scenario. What happens when we get deep into a 12-play drive? What happens if our defense has to go on the field after a 3 and out? What about mental toughness?!" Blah, blah, blah. I'll concede there is a grain of truth to this:

Only preparing athletes for the average scenario does not optimally prepare them for the less ordinary periods of extended work, limited rest, or higher reps they will undoubtedly encounter at some point throughout the season, and which arguably are of greater significance to game outcome. There is also limited psychological benefit to being used to being extremely fatigued and uncomfortable but still executing.

However, coaches must be mindful of extrapolating so far beyond typical game scenarios that they begin to prepare athletes for their ability to meet the demands not just of a worst-case scenario, but a never case scenario. For context the longest drive in college football history stands at 26 plays. No team in college or professional football has come close to exceeding this figure in 15 years, and the play count does not account for player rotation and lengthy stoppages such as media, official timeouts, and team timeouts.

The worst-case scenario is grossly overstated in most instances, and represents a minority of what athletes are doing for most of the year. Focussing exclusively on this at the expense of the typical game demands is counterproductive. For example, excessive glycolytic "train till you puke" activity significantly impedes the development of speed, strength and power. There is a small place for such training, but it has a short window of adaptation, and is incompatible with many other aspects of training. As such it should represent the frosting on the cake, not the cake itself.

GPP vs SPP

In looking at testing data and conducting the thought experiments described above, it can be easy to succumb to the notion that just because a given movement, quality or pattern of activity is not "specific" that it can be discarded altogether. Just because it is general does not mean it isn't useful or important. Linemen may occasionally need to sprint all out in a game. Wide receivers may occasionally need to block. If the lineman has done nothing but lift weights and the receiver has done nothing but sprint "because specificity", the end result is likely a torn hamstring and getting flattened respectively.

To be clear, general activities can have a powerful impact on the programme, either in laying the foundation for or mitigating the risk of more specific qualities or activities down the line, by taking advantage of the trainability of young athletes so that we can keep the ace of SPP up our sleeves, or for ensuring the necessary sporting foundation for those rare occasions when athletes are asked to do something out of the ordinary in training or competition.

Both general and specific training means should continue to be present throughout every stage of the athlete's career or competition calendar. But the closer you get to the business end of the year (the season) or career (college starter or pro), the more specific training matters and vice versa. This is the stuff that separates elite from good and good from poor, so it cannot be neglected at the expense of training for stuff that has no predictive value for the sport.

Development vs. Expression

The nature of sport is such that the athlete has to rely on a blend of different qualities and preparations to achieve a positive sporting outcome. They have to receive sufficient training exposure to learn how to best express what they have developed in training. "What evasive strategy best fits my skill set?" "What is the best way to pace myself in a game?" "How can I modify my technique to maximise my effectiveness?" These are all questions that can only be answered via playing the sport itself. Anything else lacks the context or realism to achieve the desired outcome. Simply training the component pieces in isolation will not get the job done.

However, the whole reason strength coaches like us exist is that the sport itself ISN'T sufficient for optimal development of the physical qualities we know to be predisposing to success in the sport. You can't build speed when you're slowing down your movement to process information and make decisions. Simply lifting your own bodyweight or even that of an opponent is insufficient for the development of maximal strength. You're never going to display the kind of outputs that develop maximal power when you're snapping the ball every 40 seconds.

As such there needs to be a place for both throughout the year. As with GPP, development of qualities should be prioritised earlier in the career or preparation, because simply: you can't express what isn't there yet! When the foundation has been laid, the emphasis shifts to the expression of previous adaptation later in the prep or career, firstly to maximise the likelihood of success on the field, and in the case of vets, because there isn't much toothpaste left in the tube!

Fatigue vs. Freshness

If we consider the simple equation that performance = fitness - fatigue, it should stand to reason that the best performances will occur when we have maximised fitness and minimised fatigue. Unfortunately, fatigue is the currency we pay to achieve improvements in fitness (training adaptation), and these two variables tend to operate on distinctly different time-scales. Whereas some training qualities have substantial training reserves of weeks or even months, in all but the most severe cases fatigue can be dissipated relatively quickly.

Nonetheless we have to accept that in the short term, training makes you worse. For at least some time, when you lift weights, you'll get weaker, when you sprint, you'll get slower, and when you condition, you'll appear less fit. Accumulated fatigue in the short term is the price we pay for longer term improvements. Over the course of a year or career, this is an acceptable price to pay. It doesn't matter if you're a little tired or off your best deep in the off-season or early in your career. Conversely at the thin end of the wedge, where the margins between success and failure are so fine, freshness matters and we cannot justify creating significant fatigue in training if it comes at the expense of maximum performance in competition or unnecessarily high risk of injury.

As such: the further you are from games the more training should emphasise fitness (accumulation of fatigue through training) and the closer you are to games the more training should emphasise minimisation of fatigue without significant loss of prior adaptation.

Weakness vs. Strength

To paraphrase Stuart McMillan "All athletic success operates from a position of strength". It is natural that all athletes are predisposed to leveraging a particular physical, tactical, technical, or psychological strategy to solve sporting problems. What use is trying to run through people as a 5"10, 170lb receiver if you are hugely agile? If you're a 330lbs nose tackle, why try to be evasive to get to the quarterback when you can just kick in the front door? As such we have to provide ample opportunity throughout the training process for the athletes to firstly discover what it is that is their preferred method of solving sporting problems, and how to maximally exploit its use in the context of the game.

But when you only have a hammer, everything looks like a nail. Operating only from a position of strength inevitably means that your less favoured solutions or abilities can go from being comparative weaknesses to glaring weaknesses that may be successfully exploited by the opposition.

The balance must be struck in training between fixing weaknesses and leveraging strengths. As with all the other dichotomies listed above, the earlier in the career or year we are, the more weaknesses should be the focus of training. Conversely the later in the year or career we are, the more strengths should be exploited.

Physical vs. Psychological

The general rule of thumb for training is that the various forms of preparation (physical, tactical, technical, psychological) should be as complementary as possible to ensure the greatest sum development/improvement of sporting ability. For example, small-sided games research has successfully demonstrated that a variety of different metabolic qualities can be trained at the same time as the athlete is exposed to a high volume of decision making in sport specific skills.

Nonetheless, there are inevitably situations of incompatibility where one form of preparation takes priority over the others. For example, the isolated nature of sprint training is necessary to develop speed on the field but does nothing to address tactical or psychological preparation for football (other than testing one's threshold for boredom). On the flip side, most elite athletes will tell you anecdotally that there is no replacement for the occasional beasting in training- a high volume, high stress lactate bath that goes so beyond what is physically optimal that the strength coach is clutching their pearls in horror.

Both are right, and both have to feature in a well-rounded annual plan. However, we as strength coaches need to be honest that there is little if any physical difference between individuals or teams at the elite levels. Yet there exist such gaping discrepancies between teams in their execution of skill, their implementation of the game plan, and their ability to execute under intense mental pressure. These are all psychological in nature, and psychology makes the difference once the requisite physical standards have been achieved. If physical qualities were the distinguishing characteristics, combine busts would not be a thing and the strength coach would be the highest paid member on the coaching staff.

Putting All the Pieces Together

Taking into account all of the above we can define the broad objectives of a football conditioning programme as follows:

> *Athletes need to train to be able to maximise their outputs in high intensity sporting skill for about 80 total efforts. These efforts will be split up over about 9-11 total drive of about 7 plays each. Athletes will receive an average of 35s rest between plays, and about 10 minutes between drives Occasionally reps per drive, and intra-rep and intra-set rest periods may be reduced to reflect worst case scenarios (with the understanding that eventually this detracts from the ability to prepare for typical case scenarios if trained excessively long or taken to extremes)*

Throughout the year there should also be a transition from more general training to more specific training, from addressing weakness to exploiting strength, from developing adaptation to expressing it, from chasing fitness to managing fatigue, and from physically prioritized training to psychologically oriented training in the event of conflicting training objectives.

Reverse Engineering

Just like any journey, now that the "final destination" of a conditioning plan for football has been established, we need to work backwards and navigate from where we are now to where we want to be, striking the most appropriate balance between expediency and safety that we can muster.

I have found an adapted version of funnel periodization by endurance coach, Renato Canova, to be the best way to achieve this. Funnel periodization basically re-states what we discussed above: simply operating at game/event speed while great for rehearsal and expression is insufficient for optimal physical development. It isn't until we operate above and below the speed of the event that we begin to stimulate the kind of adaptations that underpin performance but are not sufficiently developed by the event itself. (*In the interests of brevity, I will speak only about the activities occurring above game intensity as it pertains to football in this piece.*)

Adapted to football: we can all agree that the time motion demands of football are loosely those of repeat sprint/high intensity activity, and somewhere in the middle of our absolute capacity. Football isn't maximal by any means due to the short rest periods and decision-making components, but it certainly isn't a low-level aerobic activity either.

The research has shown that limited volumes of dedicated repeat effort conditioning are indeed useful for improving performance, however this is not a long-term productive strategy because none of the underlying physical qualities like maximal speed, aerobic capacity, or glycolytic power or capacity receive a sufficiently focussed training stimulus. To reflect the specificity and limited shelf life of such training, my preference is that it represents the final conditioning block of the year before training camp (July), and lasts a few weeks. Ideally this block would occur during camp, and I would collaborate with coaches to devise practice scripts to create these kinds of work conditions. However, I am a realist.

Working backwards, we also know anecdotally that the number of efforts, the sprint and acceleration distances, the accel/decel counts etc. in a game tend to greatly exceed what optimally develops maximal output in high intensity actions. For example, it is not unheard of for a dedicated special teams player to rack up more than 20 sprints in a busy game with a lot of kick off/return and punt/punt return plays. I have yet to find an athlete who can sustain >95% of their max output in a speed session for this number of reps (half that if I am lucky), even with full recoveries, so there is clearly a disconnect here between what the game can demand and what we know is ideal in training.

The implications of this are twofold: firstly, athletes will probably break if we don't gradually build them up to the kinds of worst-case scenario volumes we see for high intensity game actions. For this reason, my preference is to spend the bulk of June and the early period of July gradually accumulating volume in these efforts.

Second, the longer we spend operating at these kinds of volumes, the less likely it is that we are actually developing maximal output in high intensity game actions. As a result, there has to be a dedicated period of "optimal" training prior to this, characterised by lower volumes, longer rest periods and higher intensities. My preference is to make this training block as long as possible because these qualities are simply so stubborn to develop, and because their development offers far more indirect benefit to performance than other blocks: output for its own sake, increasing conditioning indirectly via performance reserves, and offering less interruption to the development of tactical-technical preparation e.g. install, and lower level aerobic ability, both of which tend to suffer when you are awash with lactate in later blocks. Typically, I will dedicate at least all of May and some of June to this block.

Lastly, we have to accept that training to develop maximal output entails a degree of risk. If the necessary foundation of technique, tissue robustness, and work capacity is not developed first, high intensity training can result in unnecessarily high risk of soft tissue injury. Consequently, the first training block after spring ball is dedicated to just this. In this block, intensity is managed via reduced movement speeds in the form of additional load, reduced rest periods and occasional sub-maximal effort. Is this truly above game speed? Does it fit neatly into the concept of funnel periodization? No, but it works. If you're finishing spring ball in March, this block should be conducted during April. If you're not finishing spring ball in March, you should be. Spending months to peak for a game that nobody cares about, and eating into your prep time for the games that do matter is a fool's errand.

Working Forwards, We Arrive at the Following

The Annual Plan

Month	High intensity conditioning focus
April	Prep to mitigate risk of max output training
May to mid-June	Optimal volume/intensity to develop max outputs
Mid-June to mid-July	Accumulation of high intensity efforts to game volumes
Mid July to training	Repeat high intensity efforts/worst case scenarios
Training camp	Speed top ups and survival

During training camp and the season, all high intensity field work is dedicated to football with the exception of extremely low dosages of maximal speed work to ensure hamstring robustness. Research and anecdotal experience have demonstrated to me that the stop-start nature of the sport is more than sufficient to retain acceleration ability throughout camp and the season, but that top speed needs direct training. All other conditioning work is achieved either indirectly via football for the high snap players, with limited additional tempo running work performed by low snap and non-selected players, though the details of this work extends beyond the scope of this piece.

This above process can also be repeated for spring ball albeit in a truncated fashion. This should not be as much of a concern as in the summer as NCAA practice limits place a natural constraint on just how much damage we or the coaches can do. However, as with any time throughout the year I recommend working closely with coaches to carefully manage the content, intensity, volume, and frequency of practice once practice has resumed, and to work diligently with your athletes to ensure as much work as possible is done during December and January prior to arrival on campus to negate the need to rush to get ready. Despite what sport coaches would like to believe, there are hard limits to what the body can achieve. A dedicated woman can't try twice as hard to have a baby in 4.5 months, you can't sleep faster, and peak condition for football cannot be achieved in a few weeks.

Weekly Plan

I have had great success in implementing a Charlie Francis style high-low training split as it pertains to preparing for football. When we start out there is of course not a huge deal of difference between high days and low days- we've simply not earned the right to hit true highs yet, nor generated enough fatigue to merit true lows to recover from it. It isn't until the later months of the prep that there is a true difference. Regardless, we have clear differentiation between days where we do harder, more intense stuff and vice versa, with the high days being separated by at least 48-72 hours. This means that in any training week there will be a maximum of three high days per week and 2-3 (typically 2) low days.

Sprinting

Given that football is primarily a running based sport, I dedicate two of these high days to sprinting. One day each is dedicated to acceleration and top speed respectively in terms of the teaching and also the sprinting where appropriate. These two sprint days are scheduled on Tuesday and Saturday, to provide as much rest time as possible between sessions for the lower body, especially the posterior chain.

In the prep phase, all sprint work is performed on a hill with walk back recoveries. Once the prep phase is complete, we will conduct sprints on the flat, progressing in a short to long fashion. Linemen are capped at 20yds to manage the risk of such large athletes operating at top speed. Everyone else is capped at 40yds. Once these speeds/distances have been achieved, we will split the focus of the speed sessions: one day of accelerations (prowlers for the bigs), one day of fly sprints and gear changes (unresisted accels ≤20yds for the bigs), with the volume being progressed each week to reflect the camp/worst case scenarios. When these volumes have been achieved, we spend the final phase increasing the density of the efforts by gradually reducing the rest each week until we have matched camp/worst case scenarios.

Note: we will also perform repeat high resistance intervals a la Joel Jamieson one day per week when the speed work is finished during the high intensity accumulation and repeat sprint/high intensity effort phases. This is to further push up our number of efforts of high intensity work and adequately prepare for camp, but not overly stress the hamstrings. To attempt this number of efforts solely with sprint work is excessively risky in my experience. When we implement this method, it takes the form of prowlers for the linemen and hills for everyone else.

Agility and Grappling

The third high day of the week, sandwiched between the two speed days on Thursday, is dedicated to agility and grapple work. For simplicity's sake and to cover our bases, all positions perform grapple work even if they are unlikely to ever make a tackle or block in a game. However, the most contact intensive positions (the linemen) will perform 2:1 grapple to agility work. Everyone else will perform 2:1 agility to grapple work. You are welcome to shift this ratio according to your philosophy.

During the prep phase all agility and grapple work is executed extensively and individually with no competition. In grappling, manipulation of one's own body must precede someone else's. In agility, mastery of movement with internal focus must precede external focus and decision making. Once the prep phase has been conducted, general agility and grapple games are introduced. These are competitive in nature to ensure athlete engagement and learning, but low decision making in that the athlete only has to react, or there are tight task constraints and the outcome/s are predetermined. In the accumulation phase we continue to ramp up the volume and shift to more realistic, more decision-making based agility and grappling scenarios that more closely resemble the game, and in the final phase we increase the density the efforts while holding the volume constant.

The content of the agility and grapple games is up to you but my general philosophy is to include a broad range of tasks that cover all bases. For agility we include a variety of different movements that involve cutting primarily off the inside and outside edge of the foot, at different speeds and angles. For grappling we ensure an equal focus between blocking/hand fighting type drills (creating separation) and tackling type drills (shutting down separation) at a variety of heights and body angles. In earlier phases we also include a great deal of crawling, tumbling, and callisthenic work in the body of the session, whereas in later phases this may only serve as a portion of the warm up.

Two notes:

1. It is my experience that effective grappling and agility, while there is a significant physical component, really is driven by a strong tactical-technical and psychological mastery of these scenarios. For this reason, the major progression from phase to phase is not the force or speed of movement, but the cognitive demand and ensuring that we are providing plenty of learning opportunities to build the vision-decision-action cycle that separates great athletes from average athletes.

2. The movement velocities and forces associated with grappling are comparatively much lower than sprinting, creating far less central nervous system and neuromuscular fatigue. As a result of this, and the relative importance of tactical-technical-psychological factors relative to physical, rest periods are much shorter for these activities. Around one 5-6s effort per minute is sufficient in my experience.

Typically, in at least July and probably part of June, teams will implement 7 on 7 work. There is the strong possibility that if they are left to their own devices, players will "double dip" and repeat the high intensity changes of direction and acceleration that they were already exposed to during supervised physical prep. In an ideal world this should be measured and accounted for with technology like GPS, with structure provided to the staff and players about how to manipulate the loading parameters of the session to achieve physical objectives at the same time. Unfortunately, I've only seen this done once (congratulations, Purdue), so your best bet is to just get it done on your own time and cross your fingers.

Regardless, there is almost a zero chance that any grapple specific or contact prep work is getting done outside of dedicated physical prep time. This should be alarming to everyone involved as the current NCAA "acclimatization" policy only mandates two days of helmets, and two days of shells, before full pads and 100% contact and intensity is deemed appropriate. There is no quality- physical or otherwise- that can be ramped up from zero to one hundred percent in less than a week. As such we have a moral duty to our players to be exposing them to grapple/contact work prior to camp. Label it however you like to get around the NCAA regulations. The irony is that the regulations, as written, are actively putting players at risk.

Individualisation

This overview reflects the constraints of the environment it was developed in, namely FCS Division1 football. If you have worked in this setting you will probably already be aware of the typical challenges presented, including but not limited to:

- NCAA regulations that limit the amount and nature of contact hours coaching staff can have with athletes.

- Limited resources to track workloads, diagnose training needs or monitor training intensity.

- Scheduling difficulties as a result of academic and work commitments.

- Lack of integration with sport coaches and medics due to a combination of education, ability and resources.

As such the structure of this programme is not ideal, but what we could make work with the time, staff, resources, and administrative support we had at the time. Nonetheless, we were able to record substantial increases in conditioning as evaluated by our proprietary conditioning test (The Tribe Test) throughout every phase of the year, despite utilising minimally dosed sprints, tempo runs and football practice for the duration of the season.

It is possible that you do not face as many challenges, or you face a different set of circumstances altogether. Perhaps you work in the pros where instead of the NCAA regulations, you are forced to navigate the NFLPA collective bargaining, and the tight relationship many players share with their private sector trainers. If you work in the high school setting it may be that you have much more freedom with regard to the content of your sessions, but you lack time.

In any event, the objectives and underpinning principles of effective conditioning for football do not change, only the cost: benefit decisions we make to achieve them. Ask yourself:

- What qualities does the game demand? What does success look like?

- What are the constituent pieces that underpin the expression of these qualities?

- What is the current status of the athlete/s?

- What specific factors on the ground do you need to account for in formulating your plan- equipment, space, time, team culture, athlete preferences, your own strengths and weaknesses etc.

- In consideration of the above, what training interventions can be implemented to address this discrepancy most efficiently to result in the greatest sum development of the aforementioned qualities?

Testing

The intricacies of testing are worthy of an entire chapter in itself but to my mind testing should fall into two broad categories- those which most predict readiness to compete in the sport or position, and those which most inform training decisions. Frustratingly, these two categories tend to exist in opposition to one another. A Montreal track test may be fantastic for inferring VO2 max accurately, inferring a deficit of aerobic development, and prescribing MAS intervals in subsequent training, but it completely sucks for predicting who is ready to meet the time motion demands of football.

On the other hand, a maximally explosive, intermittent repeat effort test that closely replicates the time-motion demands of football is likely to much more accurately predict who will be ready to play or be productive in football. Unfortunately, such a test is likely to heavily tax all three energy systems to varying degrees, require high mechanical efficiency, and high central nervous and neuromuscular drive. In summary, you'll know how well they did, but not why they did it or what to do about it.

In an ideal world, you would pick two or more: one to understand how well they did, and one or more additional tests to dig a level deeper and understand where the limiting factor within the system might be so that targeted interventions can be developed to maximise the return on invested training time and effort. Unfortunately, most teams are forced to pick, and we were no different at the College of William & Mary.

Given our relative inability to individualise training due to staff and time constraints, we opted to replicate the time-motion demands of football as closely as we could, and adopt a utilitarian approach to training: the best programme for the largest number of athletes, most of the time. In researching the time motion research regarding football (cited previously) and football specific tests, we were surprised to find that none existed. So, we decided to create our own: The Tribe Test.

In short: we devised an intermittent shuttle test. Athletes have 5s to sprint out from the goal line to the 20yd line and back (covering as much distance as they can) in 5s. They have 25s to walk back and recover before the next rep, and they perform 12 reps total. The distance covered for each rep is measured, and added together for a total distance score. We found it to be extremely effective and time efficient, and it has received a great deal of attention within the football community, including at the 2019 NSCA Coaches Convention. If you would like more information on this test, a full hour presentation is available on the Strength Coach Network YouTube channel.

Who is Keir Wenham-Flatt?

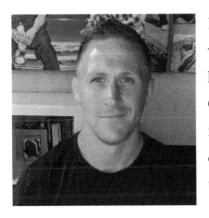 Keir Wenham-Flatt is a strength & conditioning specialist with over a decade's experience of working at the elite level of sport in 5 different countries. As part of Strength Coach Network, Keir works to provide educational, networking and career resources of strength & conditioning professionals of all levels from some of the world's best coaches.

4

Digging Deeper with Your Data

An Argument for the Law of Parsimony

Dr. Bryan Mann

So many times, as a younger strength and conditioning (S&C) coach, I did tests just because you were supposed to do them. I didn't ask questions, I didn't ask about interactions, I didn't ask anything. I did what I was told, I tested the athletes on standard tests and I looked for improvements. As I started to get older, I started to question why we did what we did, and why were we doing these things? During this period of questioning, I began doing some serious literature reviews (some call it research, but that's for an entirely different article or book) and noticed- with many of the tests that I was doing, I was only getting a small fraction from them compared to what I could. There were so many prediction equations, it was crazy how much more information there could be derived. With the use of simple equations we can go so much deeper with the data we normally collect.

Whenever we look at our testing data, we only see the surface. We see times, distances, weights, reps, etc. That's it. But when we combine prediction equations with the data we already collect, we can go so much deeper into training adaptations and what the individual needs. I remember the stories of people protesting Black Sabbath, saying that they shouldn't be on the radio waves or allowed to perform because they were satanic. I remember reading about them saying war pigs was a satanic anthem. When I heard this, I was young, and Ozzy was the prince of darkness, so I took it as gospel. Later though, in my late teens or early 20's, I heard war pigs again. I didn't know that it was Black Sabbath, nor the song. I just thought it sounded pretty cool. I looked up the words, and then everything clicked. This was the band I'd heard about in my childhood and decided not to listen. These lyrics, though, were not satanic at all. Yes, they used some dark allegory, but it was a war protest song. They were protesting the people running the machine, using the lives of common people to facilitate increases in their bank account. Just like war pigs had a deeper meaning, so too can the data you are already collecting.

Deeper with the vertical jump:

Here is a story that I have told many times, if you've heard it before, my apologies. We had a student athlete who was recruited as a safety, he was a bit of a late bloomer in terms of growth, and he grew a bit taller and wider his senior year. When he got to campus, they were thinking about trying him at outside linebacker. As college students often do, they go a bit crazy when they are no longer under their parents control of what they eat. He had found a small local pizza place that had good pizza, massive serving sizes, and was quite cheap. By the end of his first summer he was an inside linebacker. By the end of his red shirt year he was a small defensive end, and then eventually a 300lb defensive tackle. As you would expect, his vertical jump decreased during each testing period. As his position coach was a bit of a numbers junky, he was berating this athlete. His vertical jump had declined in every testing session, as seen in Table 1. He had experienced a five-inch decline in his jumping performance.

Date	Jump (inches)
June 2002	36
August 2002	35
August 2003	33
August 2004	32
August 2005	31

Table 1. Vertical jump heights for the football player in question.

I can understand the coach's frustration. When we examine the vertical jump alone, it does appear as if the player must not be putting in the work expected of him. Otherwise, why would he have experienced such a steep decline? This is not to say, of course, that his vertical jump was subpar. If you examine defensive tackles in the NFL combine, if someone jumps 31", they are recognized for having good jumping ability. So, while he can no longer jump as high as he used to it appears to represent a poor work ethic. However, his jump height did appear to also have him at the upper end of the spectrum of abilities for players who were selected in the draft for his position.

Having worked with this athlete a great amount, I knew that slacking off was not in his vocabulary. If you have additional mass, it will be difficult to jump as high as you did when you were lighter. For instance, go do a vertical jump and record the number. Go and grab a 20lb weight vest and repeat the test, you will not get as high of a jump. As long as there has been easy access to force plates, researchers have derived equations for different populations to be able to estimate power. For the vertical jump, it appears to be quite simple. Most of the equations simply use jump height and bodyweight to derive the equation. I chose the Sayers equation (4), mostly because he worked at the university, and he and I were working on a project together.

PAPw (Watts) = 60.7 · jump height(cm) + 45.3 · body mass(kg) - 2055

When I placed all his data into Table 2, it became clear. Yes, his jump had decreased over time, but his total power had gone up drastically.

Date	Weight (lbs.)	Jump (inches)	Power (Watts)
June 2002	180	36	7201
August 2002	215	35	7768
August 2003	255	33	8283
August 2004	280	32	8644
August 2005	305	31	9004

Table 2. Vertical jump height, weight and power for the football player in question.

As can be seen, this player had seen an increase of over 1800 watts during this period with a five-inch decline of his vertical jump. One must ask themselves, who would they rather have playing defensive tackle on a NCAA Division 1 BCS football team, a 180 lb. player jumping 36" and producing 7201W or a 305 lb. player jumping 31" and producing 9004W. A quick scan of the rosters will show that there are no 180lb starting defensive tackles at the Division 1 level, which automatically makes the 305 lb. player more valuable.

While this is an extreme example, this is an excellent one of doing more with your data. Some individuals lack context and think that jump height should always go up as a positive result of training. Why the jump went up is what should be examined. Sometimes an increase in jump height comes as a result of weight loss. As the height of a vertical jump is dependent upon the speed of center of mass upon takeoff, a lighter person can generate more momentum more quickly, leading to a higher velocity and thus a higher vertical jump. If a person gains muscle mass they have gained weight, they may not be able to overcome their new mass as quickly and have a lower velocity, resulting in a lower jump height.

The use of power may be a better indicator of performance over time as it will also account for bodyweight changes that occur over time. Weight gain will occur with both physical maturation and resistance training; it may be good to see if the changes in mass were functional. We can also go a bit deeper if we want to examine the relationship of allometrically scaled power. While this is an oversimplified way of saying it, allometric scaling allows one to examine all of the athletes simultaneously and look at the changes of contractile tissue. Allometric scaling most commonly uses a 0.67 exponent for bodyweight. This accounts for skeletal tissue. Skeletons do not scale in their proportions. This means that the skeleton of someone who is 5'6" has a smaller mass than the skeleton of someone who is 6'6", thus simply dividing by bodyweight gives a major favoritism to the 5'6" individual as the 6'6" skeleton has to be heavier to account for gravity and the ability of the levers to pull. Using allometric scaling; you can see who, pound per contractile pound, is the most powerful.

Deeper with the Data: *Conditioning tests*

While many conditioning tests vary in what they can find, there are a few things we can get from every conditioning test: of course, their results on the conditioning test, indicating passing or failing, a maximum heart rate and a heart rate recovery score, and most likely an anchor to use for RPE scores.

For heart rate, many of us fall back upon the default 220-age. This is fine, but can greatly lack accuracy, which impacts the validity of the training impulse (TRIMP) scores. 220-age has a standard deviation around 10 beats per minute. Why would anyone estimate the heart rate with something that can be off by so much? Simply, because it is a good starting point. I often remind people that mean data is an average, and one person can throw that average off. There is an old statistic joke that the statistician drowned in a lake that had an average depth of 2 inches. He happened to step into the hole that was 12 feet deep, while the rest of the water was at a depth of 1 inch.

It is not a problem to estimate but realize that you can be off by a significant amount. As many teams are already collecting data on heart rate using chest straps, it would be a wise idea then to simply take the maximum heart rate during the conditioning test and use that for the maximum. This would be considered a direct measurement as opposed to an estimate, which has inherent error. By using the maximum heart rate during the conditioning test, you are ensuring the integrity of the heart rate data.

However, we may need to go one step further in this example. Many heart rate systems use the heart rate reserve method with the Karvonen equation, as opposed to the traditional 220-max. The reserve is determined by maximal heart rate - resting heart rate, this essentially considers the person's current condition - the difference between resting and maximal. This method also has the advantage of being able to be interchangeable with the VO2max prescriptions. Most computer software will simply use the average resting heart rate for healthy American's - 60 beats per minute. I bring this up because I found this out the hard way. I believe I was still using the Polar Team 2 system (but it is entirely possible it was the Team 1, I used both). We had entered in all the maximal heart rates using the 220 - age formula, and when we were doing the conditioning tests, some of the athletes' data just didn't compute with what I was looking at in terms of facial distortion and posture. Then when I looked at the system, I realized that what I would see during a conditioning workout and the conditioning test may well be higher than what I was seeing on the predicted formula. This made a drastic difference in the TRIMP scores and was closer to matching the eyeball test. Then I noticed the resting heart rates and how they were off, everyone was 60. So, then I decided to bring the entire team in and perform a resting heart rate. I gave up a lifting session (6am) and instructed the students to come in but have no caffeine or any other form of stimulants. We then had them lay down in the dark and allowed them to get comfortable and essentially lay there and fall asleep. We pulled the resting number as the lowest heart rate during this period. After this, the TRIMP scores became in line completely with what I saw. So, what is the takeaway here? Know the how, what, when, where and why of what you are working with. I made mistakes for about 12 months before slowing down and figuring out the issue - it was not the technology, but my lack of understanding with what it was using that was the problem. After we settled these issues, it was a great benefit to us.

Now, back to the point of the chapter. As mentioned previously, it is far better to measure maximum heart rate than it is to estimate it. The conditioning test should be the hardest task that the athlete will do, therefore a heart rate max should be achieved during this event. If it is not, it indicates that either the person did not put out full effort during the event or they were not challenged by the event. Either circumstance would seem to make the impact of this variable moot as it would discredit the validity of the test. So, during the conditioning test, provided it is a valid conditioning test, the person should achieve a true heart rate max. Simply record the maximum number displayed from the software as their heart rate max as opposed to their 220-age number. To say that you should never do 220-age is a fallacy as well, as it is better to estimate with something rather than to go at random. HOWEVER, if you're going to be performing the test anyway, you should replace the estimated heart rate maximum with the tested heart rate maximum.

Another factor that can easily be taken from a conditioning test is heart rate recovery. After a conditioning test is performed, the athletes typically endure a period of passive recovery. By examining their heart rate upon completion of the test to 1- and 2-minutes posttest, you will be able to examine their maximal heart rate recovery, as it is the difference between the moment they crossed the line and then the 60 second and 120 second interval. It has been argued by some practitioners that the heart rate recovery should be the actual criterion for passing the conditioning test rather than the ability to complete the test. The practitioners felt that many athletes simply will themselves to complete the test. While they would be under-recovered for several days after the test they had completed as a part of their participation with the team and could continue with play and practice. However, they would not be able to fake their physiology. The practitioners argued that if the athlete's cardiac system was unable to recover posttest, this indicated that they were not in good enough condition to practice and participate in the sport.

During some of the conditioning tests, there is also the ability to derive further information such as maximal aerobic speed (MAS) and VO_2max. For each test, it will of course have its own individual equations to estimate/predict from the data taken during the test. For instance, with the 30 –15 Intermittent Fitness Test (30 –15 IFT), the MAS score is simply the last stage that you successfully concluded. So, if you achieved a score of 17.5, that means that your MAS is 17.5 kph. If you divide kilometers per hour by 3.6, this gives you a MAS in m/s, which is the unit that most coaches tend to base their programming on. Through the use of equations accounting for gender, age, body mass and 30 –15 score, a VO_2max can be estimated as follows (2);

$$VO_2max = 28.3 - 2.15(G) - 0.741(A) - 0.0357(BM) + 0.058(A)(VIFT) + 1.03(VIFT)$$

where A is for age in years, G stands for gender (1=male, 2- female), BM stands for body mass in kg, VIFT is the score of the 30 –15 IFT.

From this test, you can find the MAS, Max HR, HRR, and VO_2max. While there are other variables that can be computed from this test, they are not necessarily commonly used variables, and thus were not reported here.

For any conditioning test that you do, that has been validated, it is likely that there will be equations to at least derive MAS and VO_2max. A simple google scholar search with the appropriate terms will yield what you are examining. For instance, the Čović paper cited (2) was found by entering 30 –15 IFT score and VO_2max.

As mentioned in the vertical jump example, athletes change bodyweight quite often. In a study examining one cohort of college football players, they changed body mass, lean mass, and fat mass on an annual basis, with each year being statistically different than the other. It can be assumed that for many sports a similar relationship exists. By calculating VO_2max you increase the likelihood of seeing an actual change in condition as opposed to a change in ability to perform the test which would account for changes in body mass. This would allow you to examine if the program worked to enhance aerobic capacity despite the changes in body mass.

Now for the rating of perceived exertion (RPE). RPE is something that has been used by researchers and practitioners for a long time. Often times it is lauded for its subjectivity, when given an anchor the objectivity becomes greater. An anchor is simply a reference point so that the individual understands what constitutes a 10/10. Conditioning tests are usually what is considered the hardest thing someone will do all year, which would correspond to the 10 which is the hardest thing someone can do (6). Once the person understands what is a 10, they can then more accurately give informed RPE scores. There of course will be variation in some of the scoring, due to each individual's experience. When speaking of RPE, I usually talk about my own experience with another Likert scale, the pain scales. After my first major hip surgery, the nurse asked me "what is your pain on a scale of 0-10, 10 being the most intense pain you can take and 0 being no pain." For me, a 10 is vomit and pass out. I have been there once in my life, and twice at a 9.5 (where I thought I was going to vomit and pass out but got it under control). With that frame of reference, I answered a 4. My wife happened to be there, and knows me quite well, so when the nurse said "Ok, I'll go get you some Tylenol," she protested and advocated for me. The nurse responded that she is not allowed to give anything stronger for a 4, my wife said "do you have a scale with faces he can point at?" The nurse brought one in and I pointed to an 8. The nurse began to chastise me and thought I was exhibiting med seeking behavior. I looked at her and responded that if this is all people can handle, they're…. soft. I bring this example up to demonstrate that you often need to have visual scales for the athletes to look at. Some will understand numbers better, some understand colors better, and some will understand faces better. By giving the athletes a scale, they can identify with and an anchor, you will increase the reliability and validity of the data.

Deeper with the Data: *Squat and vertical jump*

In the Science and Practice of Strength Training, Zatsiorsky (7) introduced us to what he calls the explosive strength deficit, which is a deficit that exists between the force you can rapidly produce to the force that is not rate limited. For those who have force plates and a significant amount of time on their hands, they can easily calculate the explosive strength deficit and use this information to dictate training. However, many coaches do not have force plates, and those who do prefer not to devote training time towards additional testing. Something that I have done, but never published, is what I refer to as the power to strength ratio. I follow the same concepts at Zatsiorsky, but do not utilize the technology he did. I chose to use data that we already collected and attempt to derive additional information for the sake of parsimony. As we had already been examining PAPw using the Sayers equation for vertical jump, we had the numerator – power, albeit an estimation of power, in Watts. For the denominator, I felt that we needed a pure force metric. As everyone in the football program performed a 1RM squat, we chose to use squat with the inclusion of body mass. The inclusion of body mass was crucial to account for body weight. For instance, assume we have two people. Person A who was 340lbs and squats 600lbs and person B who weighs 200lbs and squats 600lbs. If we look at the denominators, person A would have a score of 940lbs and person B would have a score of 800lbs. By including body mass, the equations come out to be more accurate.

From this point, simply divide the PAPw by the squat + body weight. To determine what is good/bad/etc., we will have to use standardized scores, which is easy to do in excel. A quick google search will bring this up in a step by step approach. It may be beneficial to separate out groups that have different characteristics. For instance, we usually only compared the bigs with the bigs, mids with the mids, and skill with the skill. Realize that what makes the individual good at that position may pull them more towards one end or the other (in terms of a force-velocity relationship). The big position needs to have great amounts of inertia to protect the ball carrier or to combat those who are protecting the ball carrier, and thus will rely more on the force end of the spectrum. The middle positions will often have to battle with the big positions and try to keep up with or out run the skill positions, demonstrating the need for both force and velocity adaptations, equating to a very high power. The skill positions will often be jockeying for space to run routes, etc. While contact may occur for the skill positions, it is often a byproduct rather than the main intention.

For the interpretation of this variable, the use of Z scores makes it easy. If the individual is above whatever threshold you set (I usually just use +1.0), then the individual is too explosive for how strong they are and may need to enhance absolute strength to prevent injury. If the individual is below the negative threshold (I often use -0.75), then they are too strong for how explosive they are and will thus need additional ballistic exercises to improve their abilities. Here is normally where we would indicate what is good, bad, etc. However, this is a methodology that I'm not sure if we can standardize this process to what the raw scores should be. Unfortunately, there are different methodologies of taking vertical jump height (jump mat, Vertec, tape and chalk, app based, force plate, among others), each of which would bias the jump in a certain direction depending on if the method tended to over or under predict jump height. To further confound this comes the denominator, we can of course have different exercises used (squat, dead lift, front squat, trap bar deadlift, etc.) which would elicit a different number. Let's pretend though that everyone was performing a back squat – there are still several confounding variables here – depth seems to vary by institution and sometimes by coaches within the same institution, the use of knee sleeves, wraps and squat suits comes into play, the direct 1Rm testing method or various prediction methods also are in play. At the end of the day, I do not believe there is a good way to standardize this which would suit everyone's needs and desires. So, what am I saying? You will most likely have a normal distribution of your data as an entire team will have some studs, some duds, and some average people. When presented with this normal distribution, if you just standardize their scores, you are able to make accurate interpretations from the data.

Deeper with the Data: *Sprint times*

I think that we have pretty much explained time and time again why you need to account for bodyweight, as it is a factor that will directly impact jump height, conditioning tests, and, wait for it, sprint times. In a currently unpublished article, sprint times, body weight, and momentum were compared in athletes who performed sprint tests as a part of their program and were able to complete them for four years. The first and second year were significantly different, because of gaining speed. However, years two, three and four were not significantly different. During that same period, there was a significant difference in body mass, with mass increasing each year. In a study published by Dan Baker and Robert Newton (1), they investigated some similarities and differences between Division 1 and Division 2 rugby athletes (top level pro and essentially their farm team) of approximately the same age. When they calculated sprint momentum, which is the product of body mass in kg and sprint velocity, they found that while the Division 2 rugby athletes were slightly faster, the Division 1 rugby athletes possessed significantly greater momentum. As Dan has said, it is the bigger players who are just as fast that are the better rugby players. Of course, this makes sense when you step back and think of it. In my career I have had some athletes who were absolutely ginormous (6'9", 400lbs) yet couldn't move and were highly ineffective as football players. Conversely, I've had athletes who were extremely fast, but small (5'4", 150lbs) and were highly ineffective as football players. Neither size nor speed alone is the prime determinant of playing time, yet their interaction was able to separate the good from the great players.

Taking the information presented, sprint time and bodyweight over the course of the athlete's career, we calculated sprint momentums for each player. A mean difference chart is presented in Table 3. A mean difference chart examines only the changes that occurred rather than the means, essentially, we are analyzing the changes. As you can see from body mass (presented in kg), there is a significant difference every year for body mass. When examining the 40 time, there was a significant difference for Year 2 to Year 1 (subtracting Year 1 from Year 2), no other significant differences existed. There was also minimal effect on sizes for the times. When examining momentum, every year was significantly different from itself, save for a near significant difference from Year 3 to Year 4, with a small effect size. This indicates that sprint time alone may not be the best metric to track over time for an athlete's development as it does not consider all of the changes that they may be undergoing. As body mass significantly increases, this means that more force will be required to propel one down the track, which is accounted for in momentum. Of course, sometimes the only thing that matters IS speed, in sports like track and swimming. In these cases, sprint momentum may be meaningless as it has no impact on the outcome of the competition and thus should be ignored.

	Year 2-1				Year 3-2				Year 4-3			
	MDiff (SE)	Sig	d	CI	MDiff (SE)	Sig	d	CI	MDiff (SE)	Sig	d	CI
Body Mass (kg)	2.30 (0.33)	0.0001	0.13	-0.19, 0.44	1.63 (0.28)	0.0001	.09	-0.23, 0.40	1.02 (0.33)	0.002	0.02	-0.29, 0.33
40 time (s)	-0.05 (0.01)	0.001	-0.13	-0.45, 0.18	0.02 (0.01)	0.087	0.03	-0.28, 0.35	0.01 (0.01)	0.512	0.00	-0.31, 0.31
40 p (kgm/s)	23.55 (3.46)	0.0001	0.25	-0.07, 0.56	9.33 (3.21)	0.005	0.10	-0.22, 0.41	6.99 (3.52)	0.051	0.06	-0.25, 0.37

Table 3. Mean difference chart over 4 years for college football players

The great news is that sprint momentum is an extremely simple metric to calculate. If you already collect sprint times and body mass, it can readily be done in excel. I recommend changing over to metric units just so you'll actually have sprint momentum calculated. To do this, divide bodyweight by 2.2 to turn pounds into kilograms and divide the distance of the sprint in meters by the time. For instance, if someone ran a 4.74 40-yard dash at 220lbs, you would divide 36.6 m (40 yards = 36.6m) by 4.74 to calculate the velocity (7.72m/s) and then multiply by their bodyweight in kg (100kg) to get 772 kg·m/s.

Again, this interaction allows you to view the differences that exist in the athlete as they change in size and speed over the course of their career. If the individual lost 10kg and dropped 0.05 from their 40-yard time, are they better or worse? Using the previous example, let's imagine that the athlete now weighs 90kg and ran a 4.69 second 40-yard dash (this change was chosen as it is significant as seen in Year 2 to Year 1 in Table 3). The momentum would then be 702 kg·m/s, which is markedly lower than the previous 772 kg·m/s, indicating that the tradeoff for weight loss and speed was not equivalent for this individual. They do not possess as much momentum as they had previously and are not as likely to be an effective player.

In my opinion, this may also contribute to the annual "See, these college S&C coaches aren't that good," argument from the high school coaches, who often get the retort of "these high school coaches don't know how to operate a stop watch," from the college coaches. This led to a 2013 article discussing the relationship between high school and NFL combine sprint times (5). While it is true, there very well may be differences in the efficacy of the timers or from different timing systems (hand timing vs stop watch) (3), this does not account for all of it. The article specifically examined the differences produced by Braden Brown of BYU. He ran 5.20s in high school as a tight end and 5.20s at the NFL combine as an offensive lineman. According to his high school recruiting profile, he weighed 234 lbs.; while he weighed 310 lbs. at the NFL combine. When momentum is calculated, he had a momentum of 748.64 kg·m·s[-1] in high school and 991.78 kg·m·s[-1] when entering the NFL, indicating that while his speed did not improve, his momentum had increased dramatically due to increases in body mass resulting from his participation in a college strength & conditioning program and physical maturation.

Conclusion

We already collect a tremendous amount of data, at least in many programs. Before deciding that you must perform different tests, attempt parsimony. First, use google scholar as your friend. Search some of the tests that you perform already to examine what data they can estimate, for many tests, you may be surprised to learn how much can be done. For instance, if you take a resting heart rate, you can predict VO_2max, but the likelihood of this being accurate and efficacious when compared against maximum testing is low, so always take every estimation with a grain of salt. If the test is performed at maximum intensity, you can be certain that the results will be accurate for maximum intensity. Attempt to garner every single bit of information possible from the data that you already collect and are dealing with before adding in additional testing. Parsimony is akin to sustainability – if I can get the same amount of information from four tests as nine, it makes no sense to perform the nine tests. That is not to say that additional testing is not beneficial for garnering additional information, but it is to say that the additional information must be actionable.

My recommendation is to try and keep things simple. Get the most you can with the least info. Your athletes will thank you, and you will thank yourself. There is no sense in creating additional workloads for yourself that do not elicit additional info. Instead, spend that time with your family and loved ones. In S&C, there isn't enough time to see them as it is, you don't need to be subtracting from that time. Here is a little tidbit I picked up at a conference, not from the session but from the bar afterwards – keep a picture of your kid on your desk (if you have kids, otherwise significant other, pet, etc.). Will what you get from this test, be worth the time you are not spending with them? If the answer is no, don't do it. Especially not if you can get the same or similar info from typing a little equation into a spread sheet.

REFERENCES

1. Baker DG and Newton RU. Comparison of lower body strength, power, acceleration, speed, agility, and sprint momentum to describe and compare playing rank among professional rugby league players. *Journal of strength and conditioning research / National Strength & Conditioning Association* 22: 153-158, 2008.

2. Čović N, Jelešković E, Alić H, Rađo I, Kafedžić E, Sporiš G, McMaster DT, and Milanović Z. Reliability, Validity and Usefulness of 30-15 Intermittent Fitness Test in Female Soccer Players. *Frontiers in physiology* 7: 510-510, 2016.

3. Mann JB, Ivey PJ, Brechue WF, and Mayhew JL. Validity and reliability of hand and electronic timing for 40-yd sprint in college football players. *Journal of strength and conditioning research / National Strength & Conditioning Association* 29: 1509-1514, 2015.

4. SAYERS S, HARACKIEWICZ D, HARMAN E, FRYKMAN P, and ROSENSTEIN M. Cross-validation of three jump power equations. *Medicine & Science in Sports & Exercise* 31: 572-577, 1999.

5. Vint P. Comparing NFL and high school 40-yard dash times: A horrifying revelation. SBNation: SBNation, 2013.

6. Wallace L, Slattery K, and Coutts A. A comparison of methods for quantifying training load: Relationships between modelled and actual training responses. *European journal of applied physiology* 114, 2013.

7. Zatsiorsky VM. *Science and Practice of Strength Training.* Champaign, IL: Human Kinetics, 1995.

Who is Dr. Bryan Mann?

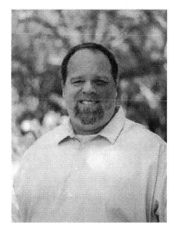

Dr. Bryan Mann is currently an Assistant Professor of Kinesiology and Sport Sciences at the University of Miami. He has been in the field of strength & conditioning at the college level since 1998. He has coached at Southwest Missouri State University, Arizona State University, University of Tulsa and the University of Missouri.

He had the fortune of working with some athletes who went on to be professional athletes and Olympians. Mann is most well-known for his popularization of various methods of autoregulation of training such as velocity-based training and the autoregulatory progressive resistance exercise protocol. Through these methods athletes are able to see rapid increases in strength and power by progressing at their own rates of adaptation. Mann has been involved in researching different aspects of athletic performance beyond just strength and power with his publication "The effects of academic stress on illness and injury in division 1 football," where they found the likelihood of injury for a starter was actually higher during an academically stressful week as compared to training camp.

Mann has been all over the world speaking on these topics and his talents have been utilized by multiple professional sporting organizations in consulting on velocity based training and other topics.

Bio from: https://www.strongerexperts.com/pages/drbryanmann

5

Transfer of Training in Fast Bowlers- A Case Study

A Comprehensive Guide for Strength and Conditioning Coaches

Steffan Jones

I fully appreciate the audience reading this may not be totally aware of what cricket and fast bowling are, so I think it is important I briefly explain the bio-dynamic, bio-motor, and bio-energetic requirements of fast bowling. It is a unique skill that demands respect from coaches and players. It is in fact, a mixture of highly stressful events rolled up into one. The closest to it would be javelin, triple jump, and baseball pitching all combined into a skill that is repeated multiple times over a long period. Lasting from 2 hours to 10+ hours! Yes, it's the 'Dakar Race' equivalent of throwing sports.

There are three general forms of the game. Short, medium, and long. The third of which can last up to 5 days. For the sake of simplicity, I will cover the shortest format. A fast bowler will cover 6-7km in total during a short format (T20) game. Based on GPS data which separates running speed into 3 velocity-running bands the numbers are below;

- Band 1: 20-25km/hr./5-6m·s/ 200-300 reps per game/2500-2700m total per game

- Band 2: 25-32km/hr./6-8m·s/ 20-26 reps per game/350-400m total per game

- Band 3: 33+km/hr./9-14m·s/ 3-6 per game/100-110m total per game

Note: I'm aware nobody runs at 14m·s (max being 12.42ms Usain Bolt) but these are the categories on the system

Fast bowlers will reach average running speeds of 28km·h (7-8m·s) in their approach towards the throw itself which is repeated a number of times with short breaks in between and peak running speed of 36-43km·hr (10-12m·s), running in the outfield as a fielder. Very few achieve these numbers to be honest, but I've had one bowler achieve 10.2m·s in the outfield. As a side note he was also the fastest 18-year-old I have ever seen. This takes me back to my argument that the fastest sprinter has the potential to bowl fast.

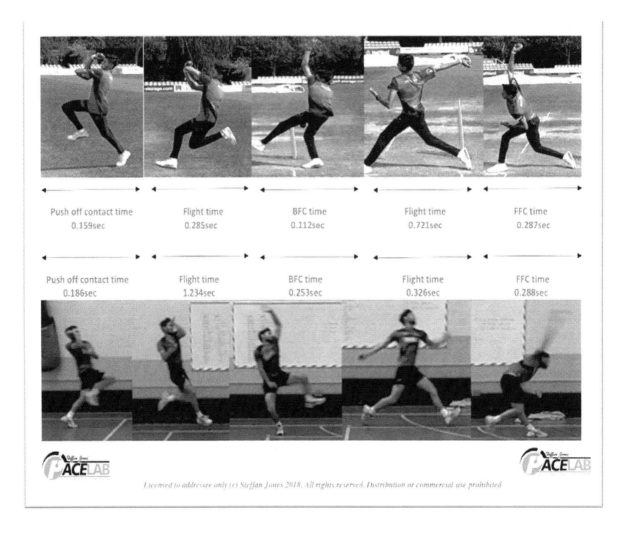

Push off contact time	Flight time	BFC time	Flight time	FFC time
0.159sec	0.285sec	0.112sec	0.721sec	0.287sec

Push off contact time	Flight time	BFC time	Flight time	FFC time
0.186sec	1.234sec	0.253sec	0.326sec	0.288sec

Biomechanically, bowling is one of the most stressful and unnatural activities you can ask your body to do. The stresses involved are immense;

Front Foot Contact (FFC) Forces: (Phillips *et al.* 2010) (Hurrion *et al.* 2001)

Peak vertical force between 5-9 x BW

Peak braking force between 3-5 x BW

Back Foot Contact (BFC) Forces: (Phillips *et al.* 2010) (Hurrion *et al.* 2001)

Peak vertical force between 2-4 x BW

Peak braking force between 0.7-1.7 x BW

And all this happens in under 0.20sec ground contact time

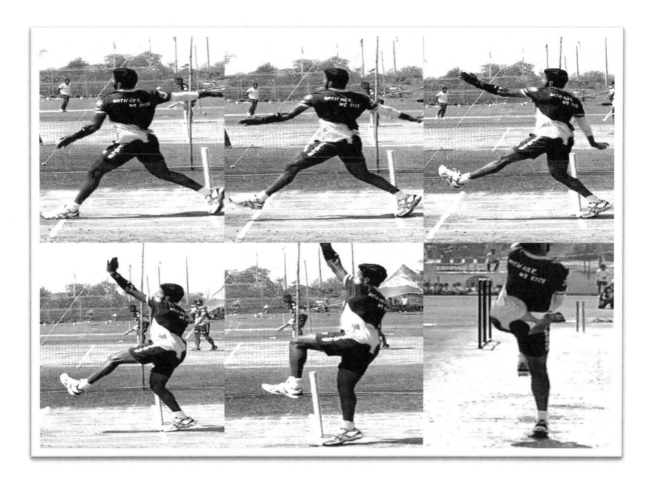

All the above depend on the individual differences that exist between fast bowlers and all athletes. It's a system I designed 4 years ago which classifies athletes into:

A. Tendon/fascia/connective tissue and hip dominant athletes

B. Muscle/contractile element and knee dominant athletes

Between each 'bowling classification' are what I call 'inbetweeners'. They can be directed towards a certain athletic profile based on anthropometry and bowling kino-sequence (technique). Their training will dictate their dominance. With all the idiosyncrasies of the human body and the physiological stresses that occur in fast bowling, training can prove to be a tough task. Which is why I firmly believe that cricket hasn't quite got it right yet. We tend to simply copy other methods that have no relevance to fast bowling. In this chapter I will explain my thought process on what is actually needed to guarantee a positive transfer of training.

The key to fast bowling is the ability to put maximum force (F=MA) into each step in the smallest amount of time. There is also mass specific force (MSF), as Barry Ross explains it in his book *Underground Secrets to Faster Running*. Peter G. Weyand and colleagues have extensively covered the topic of vertical ground reaction forces for increasing running speed, in that, "faster top running speeds are achieved with greater ground forces not more rapid leg movements".[1]

This is why you'll never be able to develop a fast bowler in the confines of a gymnasium or weight room alone. It takes 0.25sec. for a muscle to work. Based on my own research (PaceLab Ltd.) using the "Musclelab Contact Grid" it's evident that key parts of the fast bowling action happen in 0.10sec.!

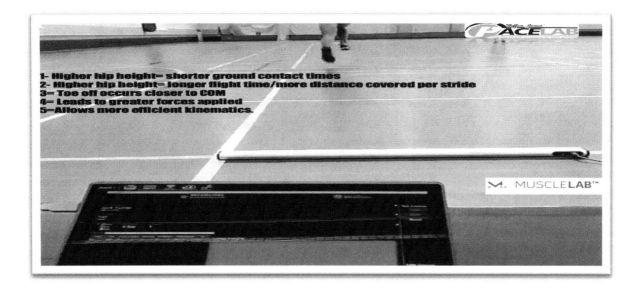

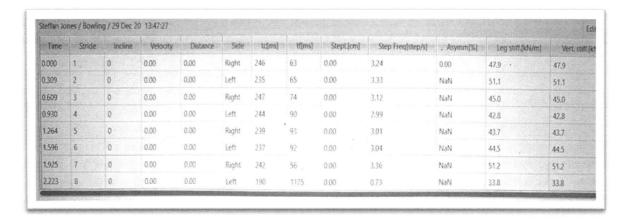

Time	Stride	Incline	Velocity	Distance	Side	tc[ms]	tf[ms]	Stept [cm]	Step Freq[step/s]	Asymm[%]	Leg stiff.[kN/m]	Vert. stiff.[k
0.000	1	0	0.00	0.00	Right	246	63	0.00	3.24	0.00	47.9	47.9
0.309	2	0	0.00	0.00	Left	235	65	0.00	3.33	NaN	51.1	51.1
0.609	3	0	0.00	0.00	Right	247	74	0.00	3.12	NaN	45.0	45.0
0.930	4	0	0.00	0.00	Left	244	90	0.00	2.99	NaN	42.8	42.8
1.264	5	0	0.00	0.00	Right	239	93	0.00	3.01	NaN	43.7	43.7
1.596	6	0	0.00	0.00	Left	237	92	0.00	3.04	NaN	44.5	44.5
1.925	7	0	0.00	0.00	Right	242	56	0.00	3.36	NaN	51.2	51.2
2.223	8	0	0.00	0.00	Left	190	1175	0.00	0.73	NaN	33.8	33.8

Steffan Jones / Bowling / 29 Dec 20 13:47:27

Not only is it about the amount of force, it's about imparting that force in a fraction of the time due to short ground contact times. In fact, less time than the muscle has to use the stored energy. SO, IT'S NOT TOTALLY ABOUT MUSCLE! Your muscles are there to support the tendons.

Transfer of Training

Fast bowling, similar to sprinting, is largely about powerful crossed extensor function at the hip (powerful reflex of contralateral hip flexion and extension) and ankle stiffness at ground contact.

> *Research has indicated that there is a very direct relationship between best time in the 100m dash, and maximal force ability within the 0.1 second window in each relevant joint to running. This shows that no matter how well-intentioned a training program is unless there is some aspect of it that is dedicated to improving specific strength and rate of force development with respect to the time constraints, results will be limited.*[2]

Athletes can do a lot of things in the weight room that happen to look like the skill itself, that don't help improve this specific 0.1 second output. The key message to begin with is understanding, "good in one doesn't make you good in the other". There are two aspects of human movement and the muscle system that need to be understood before we move forward. How much force is needed and how fast can it be delivered – the delivery system.

The Stretch Shortening Cycle (SSC) and the Rate of Force Development (RFD).

The RFD is a measure of explosive strength, or simply how fast an athlete can develop force – hence the 'rate' of 'force development'. Getting strong is about developing the total amount of force development/potential. This serves little purpose in a skill that happens quickly. In fact, fast bowling can be seen as one of the fastest skills/movements a human body can do. Arm speed of 7000d·s is registered and ground contact times of 0.09sec. during the run up and back foot contact clearly highlight this point. Nothing we do in the 'gym' can replicate it, unless it's the skill itself. That's the only true transfer of training method.

The SSC refers to the 'pre-stretch' or countermovement action that happens during typical human movements such as jumping. This pre-stretch allows the athlete to produce more force and move quicker. It's the spring effect of the muscle.[3]

The SSC can be separated into two categories based on its duration during the action:

A. Fast-SSC: less than 0. 25sec. (250 milliseconds)

B. Slow-SSC: greater than 0.25sec. (250 milliseconds)

Sprinting is classified as fast SSC, which highlights the SSC happens between 0.09sec. to 0.12sec. Fast bowling is the same. With a longer ground contact time (GCT) on front foot contact (FFC), which highlights the need for each key node to be trained differently. Back foot contact (BFC) about tendon stiffness and short GCT whilst front foot being about force management, muscle 'compliance', and eccentric strength. This is why general strength programmes simply don't work for fast bowling.

The chart below highlights the fine details and profiling that occurs in the PaceLab Training System (PST) when coaching fast bowlers. There are general and specific kinematic and kinetic descriptors that the very best achieve whilst these are underpinned by the attractors, the hard fixed skills. It is a complicated and unnatural skill that demands our fullest respect and attention when coaching.

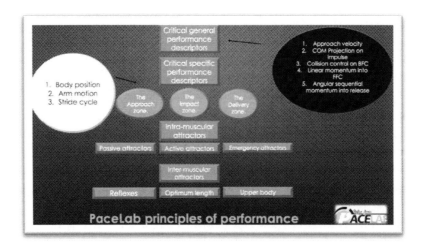

The Management of the Kinetic and Kinematic Descriptors of Fast Bowling

The training for throwing, with a straight arm overhead, and a 156g ball is highly specific and requires a unique athletic developmental program. No other sport training methods can truly replicate its intricacies. Simply using a 'one size fits all' training method is not only wrong but very unproductive. Fast bowling is very different from any other skill. There is nothing like it and it needs to be treated that way. It's not about getting stronger! Let me get that out of the way early.

> *'Problems of sport-specific strength training and the perfection of skills are closely associated with the assigned workout tasks of speed development. If the maximal strength of a given individual increases, then his/her speed will increase in movements against great resistance but not in movements with little or no resistance. Select only these exercises that increase speed in sports- specific task or technique performed with the full amplitude of movements, including the form and timing of the technique and the rhythm of the movements. Displaying speed is inseparably associated with technical perfection of movement. Proper technique permits the optimal use of one's physical fitness potential and thus high effectiveness of actions.'* [4]

As physical preparation coaches or strength and conditioning coaches (whatever we call ourselves these days), we ask our players to put their trust in us when we instruct them to lift heavy loads in the gym and to give maximum effort on the field of play. The least we can do is make all that hard work in training TRANSFER over to the playing field. Otherwise, what's the point, right?

Over the last 20 years there has been a definite focus on improving 'gym-based' strength numbers. This has given rise to what I call 'the gym white board syndrome' where athletes are trained to improve fitness tests and become top of the leader board in the large compound strength lifts. This is based on basic overload principles that some of the best strength coaches in the world are masters of. Gyms like Westside Barbell undoubtedly produce strong athletes, but they are strength athletes and not sport skill athletes on the whole. However, it's not entirely the strength coach's fault as most 'experienced' head coaches see little value in the athletic preparation world to justify their existence. Strength coaches need data to prove their worth. That's how your strength coach can prove his or her worth right? Look, I've made them stronger! There are too many variables in an athlete's performance for it to be solely come down too poor athletic preparation, right? How can you trust the tactics are right, or the technique is efficient? So, control the controllable and get their number up. I get it, I really do. That's why I adhere to 'the governing dynamics of coaching principles' championed by James Smith in his book, *The Governing Dynamics of Coaching*. Coaches need knowledge on all aspects of performance to truly make a difference.

Getting your athlete from 1.5 times bodyweight to 2 times bodyweight squat will not make them perform better in their sport. No study has ever shown this. Yes, I've read the ones which say that a squat can help acceleration when ground contact times are higher, but I've yet to read a study that says: "…if you get your athlete to power clean this amount, squat this poundage and bench press at this speed they will score more runs, score more tries, and be a more skilful player."

No, it's not out there and never will be! What we do inside the confines of a gym will never truly replicate what happens outside in sport. What we can do as coaches is to find the best solutions to replicate sport whether in whole or in parts. There has been a realization of this and a definite shift of focus in the last 2 years. With more and more head coaches searching for on-field transfer, and the realization that there is a point of diminishing return for strength to carryover due to the speed of movement in sport; strength and conditioning coaches have to prove their worth by guaranteeing a transfer of training reflected in game key performance indicators (KPI). This has led to an influx of sprints coaches and 'motor learning' gurus in elite sport and the value of "gym numbers" being questioned. Which, to me, is a good thing. The late '90s and early '00s, there was a functional training push and the 'circus training' has done a decade of damage for sports performance training. However, the realisation that the best programme is a mixture of everything, and a mixture of the methods that work for each individual in each separate sport is now advancing sports preparation training. The strength coach is beginning to be valued and respected again by head coaches and organizations.

Where players are judged, and ultimately where we are judged as coaches, is on the field. If your goal as a sport specific strength coach is to make them look aesthetically pleasing and win every fitness test, then I'm sorry, you've picked the wrong field. Your clients get judged on how many points they score and the impact they have in their sport. However, if you can confidently prove that a test score will improve performance then of course that's a different thing. This is a 'transfer of training' discussion. It's about strength isn't it? No, not necessarily;

"The real message is not that you don't do Maximal strength, or even that Maximal strength doesn't transfer. The real message is how much do you need and once you're there then what are you going to do."[5]

There's no point being physically strong and powerful if your action leaks energy or has energy blockage in the chain and the effort isn't directed at the target. Likewise, there's no point having the most clinical and 'clean' action if you can't generate enough force to bowl the ball above medium pace.

"If coaches are going to train their sprinters like powerlifters why not start with powerlifters and train them to run faster? If it's just leg strength that makes a sprinter faster, we should recruit super heavyweight powerlifters. It would be easier than the current practice of blowing up a sprinter to look like the Michelin man."[6]

Fast bowling is about force management, and training for strength is not the same thing as training for force. What is force exactly? Force is simply the exertion of physical power & can be expressed by the following equation: Force=Mass x Acceleration

Muller states that, "strength is defined as the maximum force that can be exerted against an immovable resistance by a single contraction."[7] Force can be expressed when the mass is great and the acceleration is low, or when the acceleration is great, and the mass is low.

Force= Mass x Acceleration OR Force= Acceleration x Mass

Lifting a heavy weight is an example of the 1st. The mass is high, but the acceleration is low. Delivering a cricket ball is an example of the 2nd. The mass of the ball (156g) is low, but the acceleration is very high. This needs to be at the forefront of any throwing intervention plan. Most consider training for strength synonymous with training for force, but this is not necessarily true. Strength does require force but doesn't require much acceleration. In strength training, the force that you exert against the weight must be more than the resistance you're pushing against. Realise that you can produce huge amounts of force regardless of whether you're pushing against resistance or not. In fact, the net force created by an unloaded movement can be greater than with a loaded movement. A 90mph delivery has more absolute force at impact than a heavy lift, yet the fastest bowlers aren't known for their abilities to lift big weights and vice versa.

This is why overly focusing on strength training which may potentially lead to added bodyweight (mass) may hinder your performance. Especially if you're a tendon driven hip dominant bowler. Remember their asset is the ability to be stiff on ground contact– they have springs. Adding weight has the potential to make those springs pistons, that will leave them short on both strength and stiffness. They end up with nothing! From experience getting bigger will not necessarily help you bowl faster. Maximal horizontal velocity that you can produce as a fast bowler is dependent on the amount of effective vertical force that they can apply during ground contact. The aim of every strength programme is to increase the GRF without the secondary gains of muscle hypertrophy from strength training. Added muscle bulk may not be what you're after and can hinder your bowling performance Physics doesn't care if the additional weight comes from fat or muscle if the additional weight isn't offset by additional GRF performance will suffer.

So that's why my coaching methods are more holistic. My methods synergistically combine technical work with physical work with an appreciation of motor learning and how we acquire new skills. The body is a complex system, and nothing works in isolation. As coaches we need a broad understanding and what governs the dynamics of fast bowling coaching. This is why I firmly adhere to the Bondarchuk training system.

Fast bowling is about 10% muscular and 90% CNS driven. The most important thing with the muscles is how fast they can shut off; not how strong they are. The weight room doesn't teach that, it just teaches massive, long contractions. Fast bowling is about mass specific force (MSF) in a fraction of time with correct positions that allow you to transfer momentum through the kino-sequence. This requires careful training intervention and the understanding of what actually transfers to performance.

Types of Transfer

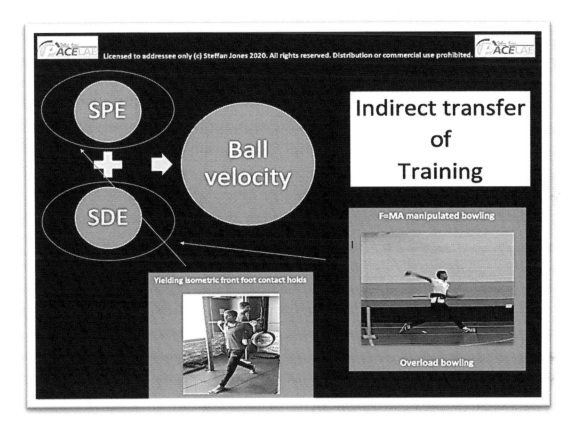

You can have *direct transfer* or *indirect transfer*. Direct transfer is when one exercise has a 'direct' impact on the performance of the competition exercises. In our case here, fast bowling and ball velocity. Ball velocity is my ultimate KPI. This is why I carry my speed gun everywhere. All 'strength' session will involve a form of bowling which will be measured. This is simply because if it can't be measured, it can't be improved. So, we focus our attention on improving the things that we can measure.

Indirect transfer is when an exercise has a direct impact on an exercise that directly impacts on the competition exercise. Still with me? An example of indirect transfer is using The Pacelab Ltd. "skill stability paradigm" (my own technical intervention system). Isometric holds on FFC to directly transfer to bracing the front leg on overloaded bowl using a 1080 sprint. Most bowlers are unable to block due to a poor management of the F=MA formula. By overloading you can manipulate momentum by slowing the bowler's approach. Take it to a place where the bowler is able to maintain a front foot block. This then indirectly transfers to ball velocity due to more effective attractor sites and achieving a specific descriptor. We know having a braced front leg helps you bowl faster. Direct transfer is improving running speed and changing the numbers on 1080 sprint approach speed. By improving sprint speed, it will raise the pace ceiling and develop a larger 'speed reserve' Your maximum speed last year is now your 80% this season. YOU RUN IN FASTER YOU BOWL FASTER. It's that simple and that's a direct transfer.

Performance and Potential

All training either produces *potential ability* or closes the gap between *actual ability* and potential ability. For example, if an incline bench press (Exercise A) develops the potential for long toss (Exercise B) with a 300g ball which develops the potential for an increase in ball velocity (Exercise C) which develops the performance you want.

If you train C, then your performance will increase up to the limits of its potential. Then you need to train B to raise that potential before you can go back to C to work on your performance again. You repeat this until B stops improving, then you go back and train A to raise the potential for B, which allows for more improvement in C. So, a basic arrangement that takes this into account would be BCBCA or BCBCBCAA.

This is the key principle of my interpretation of the 'Bondarchuk classification system'. You use the limited stimulus to get the progression you want. You pick your poison. However, you need to know what actually works which is why testing and collecting data is at the heart of the 'PACELAB TRAINING SYSTEM'–assessing NOT guessing.

You should aim to use the least number of exercises to get the training effect you're after. If you use too many you have nowhere to go after each phase. 'You've squeezed the sponge too early'. Younger athletes in terms of training age may need more variety to develop a large foundation and a bigger base to the pyramid, but spending too long in this general base of training is detrimental to achieve peak form in sport.

I believe you should aim to get to specificity in term of strength in partnership/ concurrently with a large pool of fundamental athleticism. Bearing in mind that specific strength will be more effective with a stronger athletic capacity base, but without specific strength you're just another good general athlete who fails to deliver in sports skills where ultimately you're judged. Going back to my 'gym white board syndrome!'

Training Fast Bowlers – Key Principles of the Bondarchuk System

I've previously briefly mentioned what I feel is the number one training system, 'The Bondarchuk Classification System'. Anatoliy Pavlovych Bondarchuk is a retired Soviet hammer thrower, who is regarded as the most accomplished hammer throws coach of all time. He is also the noted author of the multi-volume book *Transfer of Training*, which was translated from Russian to English by Michael Yessis and Jake Jensen.

His system serves the needs of fast bowling and my own mind-set due to the focus on improving the 'competition exercise'–the sport itself over any fitness test. Its simplicity is its strength.

My intention is not to cover the system in too much detail and in all probability my interpretation of it is different than the truest form of the system, but I've made it specific to fast bowling and my own PaceLab training system (PST). Some of what I may cover here is not the Bondarchuk system in its truest form, I fully understand that. I made it relevant to my coaching.

Rules of Bondarchuk Specific to Pacelab Training System

1. No wave loading of intensity and volume. Choose a fixed set/rep/weight scheme and stick with it. Don't manipulate volume and intensity to force adaptation

2. Keep using the same set of exercises until adaptation occurs. Use less variety. Only choose exercises that you know based on previous experiences and testing transfer to the competition exercise- 'less fluff!'

3. Classify the exercises based on their specificity GPE/SPE/SDE/CE See later for detail

4. Monitor and test every session. Follow the data

5. When peak form is hit, the whole group of exercises, called 'programme'; changes

These are the core Bondarchuk principles that bind all sport movements together, but each individual sport has distinctive nuances that are very important for sports performance coaches to understand.

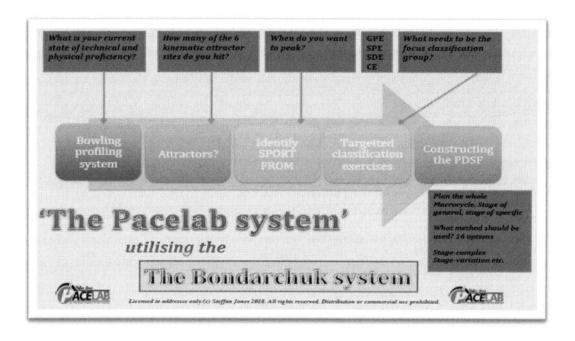

There are a number of ways of constructing the periods of developing sport form (PDSF). PDSF is the block/phase of training. The aim of each PDSF is to train the athlete to reach PEAK FORM (PF) and the exact planned time. What is PF?

The term sport PF refers to the best condition of physical, technical, psychological and tactical preparedness of the athlete. This condition occurs at the end of the PDSF. If the PDSF is composed of stages or blocks, peak condition will be realized at the end of the stage or block. The term "sport form" was initially used over 50 years ago in Soviet sport theory and practice. In other countries this condition is referred to as "top form", "best shape", "best performance" or "peak condition."[5]

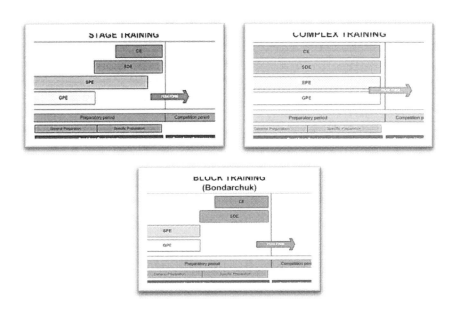

Diagrams from Derek Evely

There are certain methods that are used more often than others. Block, stage, and complex. These can be seen as the mesocycle in 'western traditional terminology'. The other methods are variation from these and in modern sport preparation involving sport and power they are heavily used. My 'go-to' as it works perfectly for the 20 weeks off season is the 'STAGE-VARIATION-COMBINATION' method. When designing shorter phased programmes, I always use a complex approach as it gets the bowler into peak conditioning quicker. The lesser the variations, the quicker peak condition is achieved. They key to the whole system is you choose exercises that will help you bowl faster. So, you need to know exactly what works! This may take a few phases of 'trial and error' to finally identify what directly or indirectly transfers to sports performance

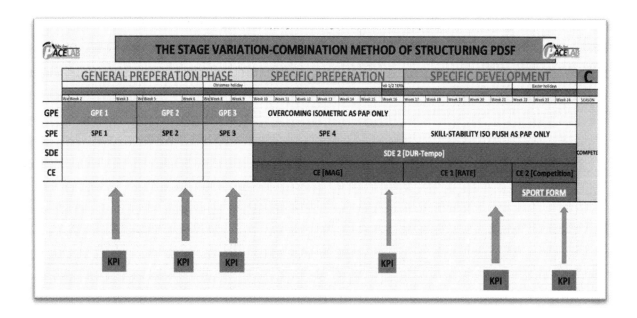

The general preparation tier can be made up of basic exercises to provide a foundation for structural integrity and support. However, ultimately every other tier is aimed at improving bowling performance. The competitive and specific developmental exercise are chosen due to the high coefficient correlation. They transfer to performance. The specific and general preparation exercise are inserted to build athleticism and injury prevention. They are there to build athletic robustness. How do you know it transfers? You have to test everything. I test every session with a speed gun. If the ball velocity isn't going up, I know the group of exercises aren't working. It's that simple. I drop them. You bring in another 'batch' of exercises but with some constants such as the competitive exercise, although that may be with a slighter different weight. Then you follow the same process. You keep doing the same programme, no variation, no wave loading, same sets/reps until progress stops. When that happens, you change the exercise group again. Only when the programme stops working. This is why testing and being 'present' as a coach is key to the system

One constant is always the competitive exercise. I'll always insist my fast bowlers bowl in their session! In simple terms choose 4 exercises, you can do a small general circuit of higher reps like 1 x 20, per session and keep them in until the speed gun tells you to take one out.

According to Anatoliy Bondarchuk to him there are actually 3 types of training transfer –*positive*, *negative* and *neutral*. Basically, I would say 80% of the bowlers out there fall into the *neutral* category, 10% in the negative category and only 10% in the *positive* transfer category. I truly believe because coaches are afraid of stressing their bowlers, only 10% of the bowlers are getting quicker. The worrying statistic is the 80% group. They aren't getting better each season. For me, if it doesn't transfer and help performance then it's a waste of time.

Early training blocks (mesocycles) whether in a year (macrocycle) or in their full career/training age are planned to give the bowler a solid foundation of potential athletic ability, strengthening their muscles and tendons to absorb large amounts of force and also teaching their CNS (i.e., nervous system-brain muscle connection) to fire efficiently and rapidly. However, as previously discussed this phase only gives them the athletic *potential ability* not *direct ability*.

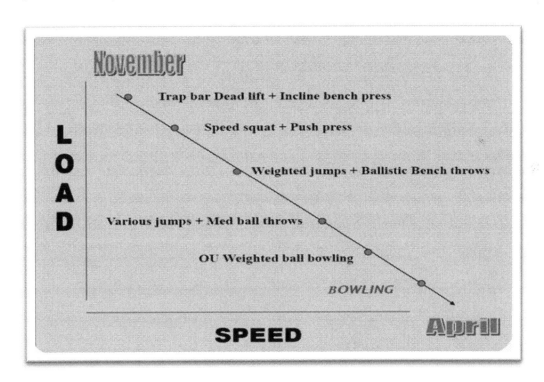

For the bowler to transfer *potential* to *direct ability* onto the field they must learn to use the newfound general strength into a quick, explosive, and coordinated bowling action. The purpose of this chapter is not to go over the finer detail of the 'Bondarchuk training system' but as it's the main principle and system I follow it will entwine itself into the remainder of the writing. Most coaches consider positive transfer of movements from the weight room, but it is fairly rare for coaches to consider potential negative transfer of gym movements, but it does happen.

The forces we encounter as bowlers are ten times what we encounter in the weight room. There is nothing that can replicate it, and please don't try to! The forces aren't due to excessive loads but due to massive amount of acceleration and deceleration action that take place when you run up, jump into gather, land, deliver the ball, and slowdown in your follow through. This is why the last phase of your winter training program has to maximise the transferability of speed, strength, and power that has been gained from hours of blood, sweat, and tears in the gym to guarantee *direct transfer*–general strength into specific strength. Specific strength is the bridge between general strength and the skill itself. It is essential and is often referred to as special strength.

Special/Specific Strength Training (SST)

The training for fast bowlers is highly specific and requires a unique strength developmental program. Simply using a 'one size fits all' training method is not only wrong but very unproductive. Fast bowling is very different from any other skill.

There is only one way to transfer gym power into game specific speed and that's special/specific training (SST). What is 'special strength?' Yuri and Natalia Verkhoshansky in their book, 'Special strength training manual for coaches' state that SST are, "Specialised resistance exercise to improve the athlete's competition performance in his/her sport discipline"

Specific strength training is strength that the bowler can actually apply to bowling. It's developed through the range of movement and at specific joint angles and speeds that are used when bowling. It differs from general strength, which is strength of the prime movers without regard for the event/skill you specialize in. It is however very important, and a phase of training needs to be dedicated to this. Having a high general strength levels doesn't necessarily mean you will bowl quicker. An athlete with a 2-x bodyweight squat may not bowl as quickly as an athlete with a 1 x bodyweight squat who has a higher level of specific strength. The athlete with a lower level of specific strength hasn't trained and transferred the general strength gains into more specific and 'usable' strength. In effect, specific strength is the bridge between the gym and the sports field. It bridges the gap between general strength work (bench, deadlift, squat, overhead press, chins) and the sporting event.

Dr. Bondarchuk states that to maximise the transfer of training gains of general strength to special strength and performance enhancement the athlete must do 2 things:

1. Choose specialised developmental exercise that are closely related to the movement patterns and neural firing rates the athlete will find in competition

2. Perform these exercises at velocities that are slightly slower (heavy balls) or slightly faster (light balls-tennis ball) than those found in competition.

Bowlers need to be bowling all year. Olympic sprinters will be running all year, Olympic rowers would be doing some form of rowing, and Olympic weightlifters would be doing some form of lifting. So why in the cricket world is it seen as acceptable to totally remove the skill from their training schedule? There cannot be a phase of more than 4 weeks when the skill of fast bowling isn't practiced.

To guarantee a positive transfer of training both strength, speed, power energy system development should all be periodically trained with the bowling sequence. Only then is it possible to achieve cohesion of fast bowling performance.

A fast-bowling program needs to do these things.

- Build specific muscles to lay foundation for the next phase

- Develop maximum strength /relative to your bodyweight (especially in the lower body)

- Tolerate high levels of eccentric stress in the posterior chain

- Develop the ability to absorb force, withstand deformation by maintaining stiffness through co-contractions and explode towards the direction of the batsman

- Develop maximum power (RFD) in the pushing muscles and rotational muscles

- Use that newfound power to transfer to game specific 'speed'

- Be able to perform that speed a number of times (power-endurance)

- Skill specific oxidative preparation ensures that the oxidative developments occur in the relevant muscles and the relevant motions as they relate to competition requirements.

These are the key training considerations that you need to consider when designing a fast-bowling program. Nothing else matters. The training program needs to be specific to a fast bowler. This is why a programme needs to focus heavily on special strength training.

However not everyone will spend the same amount of time on special strength training. What you do in a program is determined by your training age not your chronological age in my opinion.

Classification of Exercises

One of the key differences in the Bondarchuk system is the 'labelling' of key exercise groups. These are the 4 categories (classification) in greater detail;

1. GENERAL PREPARATORY EXERCISES (GPE)

These are Exercises that are performed in the early part of the GPP (November/December).

Exercises that have different movement patterns and different systems (muscular and energy) to fast bowling. Generally speaking, these exercises are very all-purpose and used whatever sport you would play. The aim is simply to make you a more 'robust athlete'. The battery of exercise is large and the decisions on what to use shouldn't take long. They are called general for a reason. High rep circuit work, prehab work, and core/trunk conditioning would sit here, along with extensive med ball throws and jumps. You would aim to perform 4-5 exercise only.

GPE exercises for a fast bowler would include:

Plane of movement	Exercise choices
Transverse	Lunge twist
Sagittal anterior	Db hammer grip curls
Frontal	Overhead plate side bends
Sagittal posterior	Bb good mornings
Rotator cuff	Shoulder sphere oscillations
Trunk flexion	Hanging leg raises
Trunk extension	Back extensions
Trunk stabilisation	Aqua bag oblique hold perturbations

2. SPECIAL PREPARATORY EXERCISES (SPE)

These exercises use the same systems (energy and muscular) to fast bowling but through a different movement pattern. They stimulate the same major groups and physiological systems used in fast bowling. For fast bowling SPE would include all relevant exercises that activate as many High Threshold Motor units (HTMU) as possible. I also use it to potentiate more specific exercises due to its maximum activation of the high-threshold motor unit. In fact, I always contrast a SPE with bowling itself. So, I contrast SPE with CE and the smaller that window between general and specific the more chance for it to transfer. Exercises selected in this classification is dependent on whether a bowler is hip dominant or knee dominant and tendon or muscle driven. Some need to 'squat until they drop", while others need to limit full squatting and actually rely on more shock training. The number one priority for any coach is to make sure the bowler is set up to land effectively on back foot contact (BFC)- the start of the kinetic chain.

However, no 2 bowlers will ever land on the back foot the same. The quality of the contact can have a massive impact on the quality of the full 'Kino-sequence' of fast bowling. Based on bowling type, ground contact times of 0.112 on BFC for a hip dominant bowler and 0.502 for a knee dominant bowler confirms my belief that bowling type dictates how they should be trained.

The amortization phase (coupling time) of the back-foot contact is critical to successful fast bowling and that the strength needed most by the bowler is not for extension/pushing off but for the prevention of excessive flexion on contact. This is a function of eccentric strength. However, understanding whether knee flexion occurs due to an ingrained motor pattern/habit or a lack of strength is really important. Some have a large knee flexion due their dominance- they are knee dominant and more often than not out squat everyone. They love the 'bend in the knee'. It's a consequence of their upbringing and their physical literacy. For example, fast bowlers in India are nearly always hip dominant due to the repetition of bowling itself with short GCT as they are growing up. It tends to be the opposite in western society. With more of a gym dominant manufactured athlete being developed and overly knee dominant. It's all about strength and movement in the knee to access the longer SSC. This serves little use in a sport where GCT are faster than the SSC itself. Fast bowling is about tendon stiffness and the most effective way to train that, whilst respecting Davis Law of collagen deposit and fascia is through specificity.

While heavy-resistance strength training ultimately produces a greater maximum force, the greater force production comes at a cost in time of application. Matching up a bowler's bio- motor strengths with their current bowling type can have a massive impact in their success and career. In the PaceLab system, fast bowlers would train their dominance 70% of the time whilst working on their non-dominance 30% of the time.

Limiting factor	Focus capacity	Exercise choices
Hip dominance	BFC quickness	Overcoming isometric BFC wall push
Knee dominance	FFC extensibility	Yielding isometric FFC hold
Muscle driven	Force jumps	Hurdle jumps/Overload sprinting
Fascia/tendon driven	Stiffness jumps	Bounding / Assisted sprinting

Based on PaceLab Ltd data, I believe there are key metric that impact performance. Along with the approach (run up) speed, the arm speed, rotational speed, back foot ground contact time, and front foot ground contact time are essential when planning PDSF's. The arm speed of an average fast bowler bowling 80mph is approximately 7000d·s/600-700rpm/36 m·s arm speed whilst rotational trunk speed is approximately half that.

A fast speed/dynamic lift like an Olympic lift which would fall into SPE. Is only 1.35m·s. A med ball throw that falls into a SDE would only be 6.23m·s. These numbers are so far away from the skill of bowling itself. So, the ultimate question would be what value do they add to a programme. So, could it just about using SPE for neural activation and efficiency and then bowling a cricket ball or under or overload balls to guarantee transfer? Fast twitch fibres are activated with 90% load or 30% load approximately (so heavy or light). Both of which don't transfer directly into bowling velocity.

For this reason, Pacelab training system does not include any Olympic lifting. If you want triple extension, maximum motor unit recruitment, do the skill of fast bowling. All weight training exercise will fall way short of what's needed on the sports field and will take time away from working on the technique that is transferable, bowling itself.

"Most lifters never get true extension before they go into their catch. They catch short so the bar doesn't have to travel as far. But the bigger issue is that a sprinter is getting triple extension off one foot and the swing leg needs to flex to get into good position. If the runner has a curved spine, he can never get into that position.

The curved spine will not allow for knee to come forward. And the neural system won't allow an explosive push when the spine is in a disadvantageous position." [8]

I hear a lot of coaches shouting so why don't you perform any Olympic lifts with your quicks? Your mind can do 3 things well, 2 things very well, and 1 thing only exceptionally well. I want my quicks mind to be concerned with one whole kinetic sequence pattern only and that is fast bowling. Olympic lifts have to be done correctly or else they are really counterproductive, stress the shoulders, and can cause injury. I'm qualified to coach it but to get really effective and efficient at it takes hours of mastering. I would prefer spending the time coaching them to become better at fast bowling and get them stronger with basic lifts in the gym.

Remember, movement slower than the actual delivery in fast bowling won't make you faster, and the lack of a negative part of an Olympic lift misses out the main muscle contraction in fast bowling. Bowling fast is all about controlling the shock and the eccentric forces on impact to avoid deformation which will increase the time to complete the sequence- not good! Faster hips can be achieved with sprinting, standing broad jumps, and overhead granny MB throws. I believe it's not ideal to synchronize hip extension with an arm pulling and shoulder shrugging motion. Fast bowling is the opposite pattern.

"Olympic lifts should always be viewed through the lens of the nature of impulse to the ground through the ankle (concentric and eccentric) when it comes to specificity." [9]

Also, remember Olympic lifts are about triple extension and coming up onto the balls of the feet. Well in fact, fast bowling is about timing of triple rotation and extension, and also BFC being on the ball of the feet whilst FFC is on the heel. The only Olympic lifting I would use is the split jerk, which is a great movement for the legs mostly. Anything "dynamic" in nature, like the DE effort day in a Westside conjugate type template is useless to a fast bowler. Weight training cannot make you move faster than actually bowling. If you need your bowler to be faster, then more light ball bowling is in order and even more heavy ball bowling.

"The better you can execute the skill, the better you can perform in the sport. Coaches have a tendency to take skill execution for granted and rely on physical conditioning as the main way to improve performance. But your physical qualities such as strength, flexibility, power, and explosiveness must all relate to how well you can execute the skills. Having great strength or power in movements or actions that are not specific to your sport skills will not make you a better player on the field! To have the best skill execution you must have the best technique plus optimal development of the physical qualities that are specific to your technique. This is indisputable."[10]

The traditional model of peaking for competition by increasing the specificity of exercises nearer competition is flawed in my opinion. I'm not saying I haven't done it, and on occasions I may still be doing it when I'm unsure of the quantity and quality of the skills/fast bowling training. My approach is very simple, **'you train in the gym what you don't do outside it!'**

'My belief is that the CNS stimulation that happens with weight training during a max attempt with max weight is greater than the stimulation during a max attempt with max power. I find the need for a maximal stretch is useless if this max stretching does not lead to a maximum contraction. Having a maximal myostatic reflex without a maximal contraction is like teaching the arm to reverse and start a movement and leaving the job unfinished. Unless the weight is maximal, a maximal contraction following a maximal stretching will lead the athlete to release the weight, thus leading to the need of bands or something similar that do defeat the purpose of weight training for throws! Because we train to accelerate a given weight and not keep a given speed for an increasing weight as leverages get favourable'- Unknown throws coach.

In simple terms you train outside competition the factors that don't get trained in the skill itself. During competition you train the factors that don't get stimulated during play itself. Training methods along the force velocity curve are on a sliding scale. When you have a large volume of one, you need less volume of another.

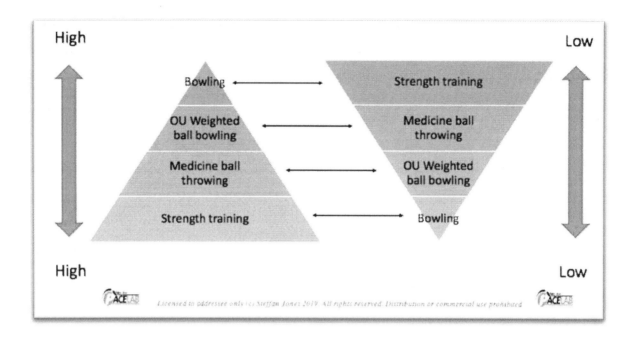

3. SPECIAL DEVELOPMENTAL EXERCISES (SDE)

Special developmental exercises use the same systems as fast bowling but are not identical. They duplicate part of the movement but not the whole movement. The speed and the joint angles are the same as a key part of fast bowling.

This group of exercise are split into different categories based on the technique of fast bowling itself. They are specific to the skill itself and serve no purpose for any other sport.

Exercise choices	ZONE 1: Approach	ZONE 2: Impact	ZONE 3: Delivery
Stiffness	Pogo jumping	Skill stability BFC iso-push	Paloff press perturbation
Force	Prowler pushing	Skill stability BFC pulse	1080 load and bowl
Speed	1080 sprinting	Assisted BFC hop + stick	Mb side throw
Eccentric [load]	Depth jump	FFC flywheel drop lunge	Shoulder sphere
Isometric [control]	IMTP	FFC yielding iso hold	Overcoming iso shoulder push
Dynamic [explode]	Hurdle jumps	FFC jump and stick	Kneeling constraints

The SDE would be categorised as specific/special strength in its truest form. These exercises look like the skill itself in some form or another. You are now using the motor potential developed from the previous tiers and combining it will the technical work that has been performed in separate sessions using methods that will increase the power output to guarantee a transfer of training and hit peak form.

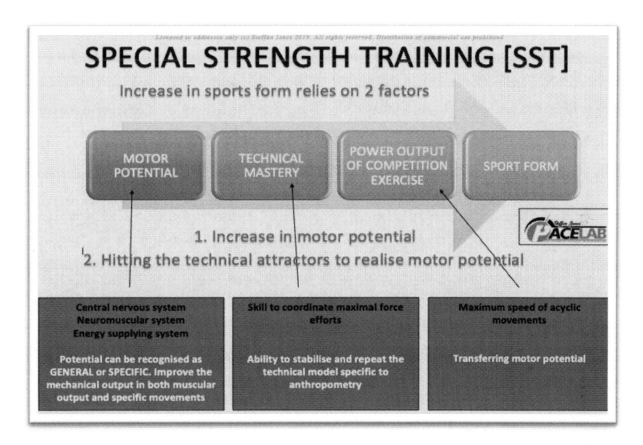

It is important to integrate the correct synergistic exercise and biomotor qualities to avoid neural confusion. Don't provide an unambiguous goal.

The Pacelab Model of Reaching Peak Form

The neural potentiating benefits of moving quickly prior to adding more force-driven strength training is something that is often ignored. As coaches we tend to just follow the crowd. Often that crowd exist in a totally different domain, a totally different spirt that in fact may actually need more strength early in the prep.

However, for me, as a coach in a skill needing more speed (80%) than strength (20%) it makes sense to move quickly first.

The closer you are to the season the less specific your gym/strength work should be. The reason you use specific strength or special strength work is to 'make up' (fillers) for what you are unable to do- bowling itself. Whether it's because you've just had a season, or the climate doesn't allow continued skill development.

Doing special strength training as well as bowling may cause coordination issues, both intra and inter muscular. Highly complex weight room movements can compete for coordination resources and also the neural pathway that can interfere with bowling itself. Another traditional approach would be to utilize more single leg exercises closer to the season and focus on bilateral at the start of the off season. This can also cause conflicting messages to the system. This goes back to my theory on Davis law and the fascia system. We need to limit the amount of overload we use that's similar to the pattern of fast bowling itself. You cannot ask the body to do everything at once especially if the message is an ambiguous one. All I say is don't rush to get to the weight room post season. Why not sprint and jump and get quicker first? At the end of the day getting quicker is more CNS than muscle and the CNS needs specificity to improve the skill itself. To avoid neural confusion when you're working high acceleration as an athlete you should be working low/no velocity as a fast bowler. I firmly believe in coaching speed before strength. This is why at the start of every new training cycle there will be a focus on developing speed as an athlete. So yes, I will get them sprinting and jumping before they squat......Stop throwing things at me!! However, this is then the same time as they develop key skill positions. Training low or no velocity but high force exercises will be used as a fast bowler. Isometric holds in the skill stability paradigm are performed the same time as the athlete is performing speed/reactive/explosive work outside on the track/hills.

The mistake coaches and athletes make is they try and make the gym training specific at the same time as the volume of competitive exercise increases. The issue here is that one method, despite being specific, is teaching the system to hold on to tension in the gym, but skill and fast bowling in particular is about 'reciprocal inhibition'. It's about creating and releasing tension at specific times. It's about the synergistic relationship between intra and inter muscular coordination

When your programme involves a high volume of the skill itself, whether loaded or unloaded there is no reason to make your gym/strength training specific. You're already doing the most specific exercise you can do.

4. COMPETITIVE EXERCISES (CE)

Purpose of every resistance programme is to encourage a permanent and positive change to performance. Positive transfer occurs when the training method replicates part or whole of the kinematic and kinetic sequencing that occurs on game day. To achieve transfer the load cannot change the biodynamic, bio-motor, or bio-energetic capacities in the body. The body must not be able to differentiate between a load that is alien to the body and the kinematic sequence of the skill if it's to transfer. This is why I extensively use a combination of weighted balls/implement and light wearable resistance suit called 'Exogen' by Lila Movement.

The only true transfer of training exercise is bowling itself. In this classification exercises are used that are identical or almost identical to fast bowling. As mentioned here the hugely effective PaceLab over/underload (OU) weighted ball programme comes in and the use of the Exogen suit. Bowlers would bowl using various weighted balls, both overweight and underweight or a fully loaded suit. All other training methods are no longer used or at best used in small volume for maintenance purposes.

I split the bowling sessions into 4 key focuses. Working on accuracy and tactical awareness, OU weighted ball bowling, tempo bowling to work on the oxidative system or max intent, run and gun session. You can only focus on two during each phase or block. Why? It's about avoiding neural confusion. Don't confuse the system. Limit what you are trying to work on and you're more likely to benefit from them. Don't try and be a sprinter and a marathon runner in the same phase/block/session.

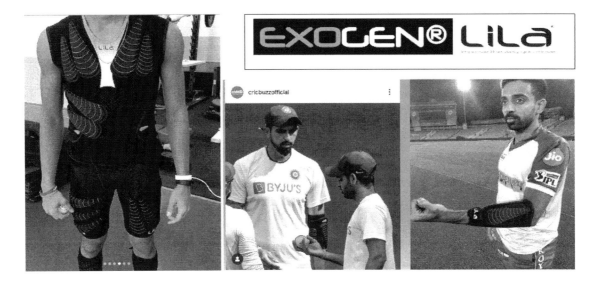

To avoid neural confusion, the combination of focus has to be periodised. Technical grooving and skill stability can be performed throughout based on individual needs.

1. Accuracy (Tactical) and intent (Rate) can be performed in the same session/phase

2. Load (Magnitude) and energy system development (Duration) can be performed in the same session/phase

Conclusion: We are Stress Managers

Constantly applying stress to the human body is the single most important component of any training program. It's fact that you must constantly be stressing the fast bowlers for them to maximise their athletic potential. This is why I believe we are STRESS MANAGERS! A coach must understand stress, its cause-and-effect relationship on the human body and how that relationship influences adaptations that help them bowl faster.

As coaches we need to understand that overloading the athlete and stressing them is key. Without it, athlete will never fulfil their genetic potential.

"Only when standing at the brink of destruction does man truly realises his potential"

Ancient Samurai Maxim

The key to transfer of training, adaptation, progression and stress management is having the knowledge to carefully plan a programme based on individual needs, sport's needs, and skill needs. Simply copying programmes from other sports is a sure-fire way of failure. I firmly believe in a systematic approach to training where planning, adaptation and progression is based on data and results. Only then can you guarantee your athlete is achieving peak form and not simply being a name and number on your own ego driven white board.

REFERENCES

1. Weyand, Sternlight, Bellizzi and Wright Journal of Applied Physiology 99: 1991-1999, 200.

2. Joel Smith, MS, CSCS. Speed Strength Manual: A Comprehensive Guide to Biomechanics, Demands and Training Methodology for Linear Speed.

3. Owen Walker. Science for Sport 23 Jan 2016

4. Starzynski, Sozanski. Science of Sports Training, how to plan and control training for peak performance: Thomas Kurz.

5. Derek Evely. EveltrakSport.com: The Bondarchuk system course 2019.

6. Barry Ross. Underground secrets to faster running. Barry Ross

7. Kelly Baggett: Higher Faster Sports

8. Chris Korfist, Extreme Speed training webinar

9. Joel Smith, MS, CSCS. Speed Strength Manual: A Comprehensive Guide to Biomechanics, Demands and Training Methodology for Linear Speed

10. Dr Yessis Ph D, 'The revolutionary 1 x 20 Strength Training Program

Who is Steffan Jones?

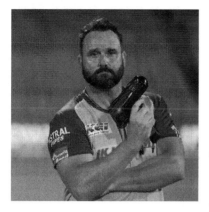

Steffan Jones is the last dual professional sportsman in the United Kingdom, having played three years of professional rugby and 20 years of professional cricket. Currently, he is the Director of Sport Performance at a private school in England and a global fast bowling consultant. He is a fast-bowling development coach for the Rajasthan Royals in the IPL as well as consulting for individual fast bowlers, javelin throwers, and pitchers around the world.

Steffan is in a unique position having played the sport, is a qualified sports scientist, a UKSCA qualified strength and conditioning coach and also as a level 3 qualified technical coach. His methods are innovative and heavily based on sports science.

Steffan has developed a reputation as an 'outside the box' thinker in all overhead throwing sports and is the go-to man when an increase in bowling velocity is required.

His focus on specific strength including weighted ball bowling, the application of the Bondarchuck classification and the utilization of isometric training as part of his skill-stability training method. It has brought him plaudits from around the world and continues to disprove the view that technique cannot be changed as you get older.

6

Transfer of Training in Team Sport

Using Technology for Testing Transfer

Jake L. Jensen, M.S.

OUTLINE

1. Test what matters

2. Evaluate practicablity

3. Test reliability of your technology

4. Examples in the applied setting

5. Evaluate transfer

TEST WHAT MATTERS – why you should read this chapter

> "A stupid fighter has no fear of death."
> - Sun Tzu, *The Art of War*

Charging into a new team, or a current team, with new technologies and a radical plan to change everything with tech is a good way to get fired. It would be like walking up to the first person you see at the rink and saying, "Hey stranger, I think you suck at your job and I can do it better than you." This strategy produces a defensive reaction in people, it's human nature. Animals resist change, especially when it walks and talks like change. As strength coaches, we can do much better with stakeholders by making the technology we are planning to deploy look like *exactly* what the team has always wanted; a solution. A healthy respect for, even a *fear* of, change can help us anticipate reactions and modify our presentation to achieve transfer.

If Sun Tzu had been a strength coach, he would tell you only a stupid strength coach has no fear of change. As we begin I want to clear the air – you do not *need tech* to test transfer. Technology can play a role here, but it is not required. This chapter is about how to efficiently integrate technology, but I am not arguing that it is a necessity. Now, we need to make effective change using technologies for our current team/organization, taking advantage of human nature. Let's talk about our three core principles to accomplish this.

Technology in sport should produce:

Perspective – Technology should give more understanding about the sport and athletes. *Understanding* is not the same as *information*. Probably good to read that sentence again. As strength coaches we have specialized understanding about developing biomotor and bioenergetic qualities. We often use technology to be more efficient with the time we have in training. Specifically, to gain higher performance in less time by focusing on developing the most urgent qualities for sport. Technology can help us to communicate this knowledge, results from training, and demonstrate our value to stakeholders. This ability to communicate makes us more useful to an organization, in working as a team with other coaches who have specialized tactical and technical knowledge.

The Rub: test only what you can. Through communication help stakeholders (including athletes) understand

Commitment – Technology should represent a journey undertaken, a promise of performance, a handshake that signals the start of *better*. Strength coaches often play the role of the gatekeeper here. This means taking on nuance with an open mind and creating systems for structural obstacles that consistently slow us down. In addition, there are moral implications here, which will be discussed later.

The Rub: test only with integrity. It's the foundation of any data driven high performance team

Agility – Technology should make us fast. Better understanding and proven integrity breaks down barriers, builds bridges, and streamlines the achievement of goals (like winning). In short, using technology makes us swift, not slow. The intent is to allow us to go uninhibited about the business of implementing the training program, and realizing its results.

The Rub: test only if testing makes you faster. Never slow the team down with data.

EVALUATE PRACTICABILITY –

Your Organization

Every organization is on a different journey with regards to performance development. You need to determine where you are on this spectrum. Many technologies have the potential to produce useful information, but organizational factors exist which will inhibit you from extracting that from your team. Begin with your area of direct influence; the gym. Does the organization have a large footprint for training or a small one? How does the flow of your training sessions dictate where or what you are able to test within that space which you are responsible for? An example here; if your gym space is far from a field, is long and narrow with barbell equipment along one wall, a 1080 Sprint may not be suitable for your space. Especially if you plan to use it during workouts to test 70 players in one session. Consider how to integrate technology into that space. Another example, say you want to test isometric mid-thigh pull, but you only have squat stands in your gym – no racks. Manageable, but you will have to create a dedicated space for this single assessment, which you are unable to train with your current equipment. In this case, a different assessment of force might be a better fit. The question becomes, how much is this "data" going to cost you in real life, outside of the expense of purchasing it? Remember, in sport we don't purchase technology with money alone, other currencies are also exchanged. Jocko Willink has said that leadership capital is the currency of teams. The cost of communication, of seeking *change* within an organization, is leadership capital. Just like coin currency, once you spend it, it's gone. We will circle back later to discuss the principles of selecting which physical qualities to spend these resources on pursuing, given your current organizational situation.

As we wrap up our area of influence, once we feel that we have maximized our ability to improve testing in the gym, we move to areas outside our direct area of influence – the tactical arena. Here we are talking about testing the game, either with displacement-based equipment (LPS, GPS, ACC, etc.) for externally derived values, or exertion-based measures (HR, HRV, RPE, etc.) for internally derived values. Additionally, you could seek out tactical/technical data to derive meaningful conclusions. Be aware here – you are in deep water. Even for the former athlete, you are in deep water. The powers that be are concerned with winning, and this should be kept in mind at all times. Quickly, and I mean VERY quickly, a well-meaning scientific pursuit can become a distraction, and get pulled up by the roots. You must consider agility – we never want to slow the team down. Let's examine testing with GPS as an example.

In this example, let's compare a pro hockey team with an NCAA team. The college kids are told to wear these GPS trackers, they do so without a second thought. They use various testing tech in the gym and have since their freshman year. Testing is as much a part of their collegiate experience as playing hockey. Coaches and directors are pleased that technology is being used to more safely and effectively develop their student-athletes. Hugely useful insights are derived from the on-ice trackers as a result of great compliance, and the players enjoy competing with each other based on the data. Relatively little leadership capital was expended in adding this measure, and it is implemented with relatively little resistance. This organization was ready for tactical testing.

Now, the pro team. Culture in this club is to purchase performance, not develop it. Not one person in the organization has a deal longer than 12 months. In fact, the gym was outfitted with only 20 bikes and a radio before you arrived. You want to demonstrate the way that strength and power influence the sport through tracking on ice. You go all in – every cent of leadership capital you have, to buy a tracking technology. You have it in hand and begin the process of integration. Rookies wear them because they were told to. Role players in the dressing room use them at first, but slowly lose interest and refuse to use them. Veterans are outright hostile, ridiculing the few players who find the data academically interesting. Coaches see this as a distraction to their mission of winning now, are indifferent to the data, and frustrated with your constant mention of it. After year one of implementing the system, poor compliance and lack of support have resulted in weak or no data – therefor no results. Management is frustrated with the weak performance you have shown after their 1-year-old investment. Now you begin to see the sharks circling in the deep water beneath you. This organization was not ready for tactical testing.

Frequency

Understand that with data, there are principles which govern what we can and cannot infer from a set of numbers. There are, in fact, rules here. As the gatekeeper, we are responsible for knowing the rules and helping our organization to avoid the penalty for breaking them. One such rule is that the less often you measure something, the less likely that measurement represents a true observation. In other words, testing more often increases your ability to make a judgement call. Think of it like a window in a cabin. If you never look outside, except for once in January, you could infer that the cabin is in an arctic wasteland, and that it never gets warm. On the other hand, if you observe the weather hourly all year, you would have a truer idea of what the climate is.

Let's bring this around to sport science now. Some qualities are reasonably tested yearly – height for example. Some are reasonably tested monthly – body composition for example. Still others could be reasonably tracked daily, such as hydration or sleep. For performance outputs, especially in the gym, we should be asking ourselves what it is that we are testing and how often can we test it. This should dictate the way we evaluate and purchase a technology. If a technology requires a barbell to be effective at testing force, ask yourself, "are all of my athletes going to be using a barbell every week of the season?" On the other hand, if a technology is wearable but requires a local anchor, such as a positioning docking center or tracking hub, ask if that wearable is going to be used daily for measurement, or perhaps only weekly. Frequency of collection matters, and should be a primary consideration when evaluating tech applications.

TEST THE RELIABILITY OF YOUR UNIT –

Don't let that word *reliability* intimidate you. This one is easy, and probably the most fun part of using technology in the applied setting. Now, there are statistical methods which are specific, require some skill to apply, and work great if you have the experience. We are not talking about statistical reliability methods here, rather practically reliable ones. Remove from your mind the answers you were given by manufacturers and sales folks. It is time to put the tech through the paces yourself. Here are a few things to key in on;

1) Is it user friendly for athletes, or do you need to run each assessment?

2) Does use integrate well into the exercises you currently use during training?

3) Try it yourself daily for a week. How widely does the data vary?

4) Finally, how well does the data answer the question you are asking?

I will give you an example here, from my experience, which illustrates the point. To answer the question of how to best develop strength and power in the gym, we test a standard counter movement jump as part our training. Now, what is a good result in a CMJ test? If you use a laser system like the OptoJump, "good" can exist within a range of 3-5cm of variability! Athletes aren't stupid, they intuitively seek to win. Tuck the knees a bit, you win at the laser jump game. So, for you as the coach, setting a performance threshold that is too narrow (say a change of 0.5 - 1.0%) for your tech is setting you up to fail. In addition, with standard variations at roughly 10% of the total performance, you may ask yourself if this technology is reliable enough to answer the questions you are asking. This is not a rigorous statistical evaluation, but it does give you some valuable reliability information about the tech you're using. Quickly, let's answer questions 1-4 with regard to the OptoJump system:

1) Very user friendly, but athletes could create dirty data without supervision (even *with* supervision!)

2) Easy to integrate into any program

3) Single efforts can vary +/- 10%. Determine for yourself how reliable that is

4) Are my athletes maintaining their power output in jumping? This tech could help me learn that

Here are a few notes I keep in mind when assessing the reliability of a new technology:

- A note on testing reliability: collecting clean data is everything in testing. A mentor of mine once told me, "you can't make chicken salad out of chicken shit." Well, it turns out some people do anyways. Messy, disorganized, unplanned data collection produces a shit-salad of confusion and frustration.

By testing the reliability of tech on your own, you hone down a collection process which cleans the data before you collect it. This is also part of your job as the gatekeeper of performance data, to know beforehand the factors influencing your tests and account for them in protocols.

- A note on validity: lab grade equipment which stands up to peer reviewed rigor is great and often requires a cumbersome amount of effort to use. However, field tests are also great, and require little effort to use. In a laboratory, using multiple force dynamometers in conjunction with EMG probes is scientifically fascinating, but useless in some applied settings. Don't forget, you are swimming in deep water. There needs to be a clear, 1:1 path to the *how* this data is answering performance questions for stakeholders. Don't chum up your swimming hole with cumbersome, confusing, measurements and bloody analysis. As you do your initial assessments, think about how these technologies will translate into performance conversations with stakeholders.

- A final note on this: just embrace the fact that you will need to do your own data analysis. The plug and play, included in the package, dash boarding tech companies provide for free is a mess. Fancy graphs and bright colors don't tell a story, and the statistical power you need doesn't exist in the black box's companies sell you. The art of telling a story with numbers requires work, and as the gatekeeper you will need to get messy, mix the paint, and put it to canvas. So, **do not expect** to slap a tracker on a guy, download the session, and print the dashboard for a coach. **Do expect** to start with a raw data set and begin mixing, before you ever wet your paintbrush to create visuals.

EXAMPLES IN THE APPLIED SETTING -

I observe five areas for testing;

Strength/power

1) Speed

2) Endurance

3) Body Composition

Strength & Power

I lump these two together because I use portable dual force plates to test both. When it comes to testing strength there are several critical elements that have to be top of mind. The mode of testing is going to dictate how well these falls under our big three principles. Using back squat, especially >90% 1RM, you could potentially alienate any athlete with contra indicators like bad shoulders, back, hips, knees, etc. In addition, questions about the quality of execution (squat depth, etc.) make things more complicated. Stake holders, such as coaches and management, rarely accept "bad shoulder" or "high squat" as a test result. So, it becomes our work to find a MODE that gives perspective, demonstrates commitment, and makes us agile.

To do this I use trap bar deadlift and key in on force production as the KPI. The exercise is virtually universally acceptable by athletes across a wide range of injury history, and the load prescription avoids issues with regard to potential technique breakdown.

Power testing is also performed on the dual force plate, using a counter-movement jump. We have gone over all the details in previous sections with regard to jumps. One note here on using a force plate system; there are some measures which are extremely variable, with respect to the origin event of unweighting in the initial drop phase. Be careful that you understand the dynamics of jump technique and how your device transmutes this into data, otherwise you'll find yourself scratching your head at widely variable, confusing numbers. The good news here, is that many companies (I use

Hawkin Dynamics) have software which control for jump phase, and allow you to bypass sticky situations like this one.

Speed

The issue here, for me, pertains to my unique sport. Ice hockey speed is not sprinting speed on grass. In ice hockey, a player can achieve a peak velocity in a time trap which (in some cases) will never be reached in competition. Thus, in hockey you end up with a peak acceleration speed and an overall peak velocity. Testing speed in ice hockey is a new frontier in where the literature ends and theory begins. So, you may be disappointed here, but this section will be short on examples. I will leave you with this; there is a potential correlation between the athletes who are fast at peak velocity and the athletes who are fast at peak acceleration.

Endurance

I have never comprehended a discipline so well objectified through physiology labs and investment, in that professional sport could be so subjective. For guys like me who have been under a barbell for the last 20 years, checking out the literature on individual anaerobic threshold is a thrill. From LAC4, to gas exchange variables, to the modes and mathematical gymnastics that produce V02 predictions, endurance is a fascinating area of study.

Tests such as the 00:30 second Wingate will likely, vastly, *overestimate* an athlete's endurance. Similarly, tests which require 40-50+ minutes to complete will definitely *underestimate* a speed-strength athlete's endurance. When selecting protocols for testing and reporting strategies for an endurance output, be sure you understand the way that the test design is affecting the numbers you report. A relative V02 max of 60 mL/kg/min in an 8:00 minute test is not the same as a score of 60 mL/kg/min in a test that takes 45:00 minutes to complete. Remember, you are the gatekeeper, it is your work to be the expert.

Currently, I use a cycling ergometer test, without a ramp. There are organizational factors at play here, such as data consistency, which influence the structure of the test. Suffice to say, it is a graded cycling test which gives me relative V02 max and an individual anaerobic threshold for each athlete. I find these data very useful, and comparison across the entire population of athletes in our club (aged 16 – 40 years) since 2016 produces a r^2 correlation of 0.6 between the two. Is that good? Not necessarily, but it is a number that informs about a set of variables, which for me is a useful bit of information.

There is work to be done on this. The bike is good because it hits multiple boxes for me. It is also good because it gives me a robust testing table to start attacking with on-ice measures of endurance. The literature on how ice-hockey endurance is connected to off-ice endurance is still opaque. If only there was a crop of strength coaches who could use technology to connect the two…

Body Composition

During my undergraduate degree at the University of Utah, I had an anatomy professor who was an absolute savage. He still works there, and has been a mentor of mine over the years. He said something that has stuck with me during our first lab session, which featured human cadavers (I didn't realize until later how lucky I was at the time) which is extremely rare for undergraduate students at public universities. The quote went like this,

> *"we could measure each of your body compositions and be perfectly accurate this way: by cutting every ounce of fat off you, putting it in a steel tray, and comparing that with the rest of the parts by weight. The only issue is that you would be dead."*

This illustrates our point here. You are the gatekeeper, and it is up to us to communicate that a measure (body comp) is just a number and has strong limitations. Body composition measurement devices exist on a scale, from most accurate to least accurate. The literature seems to classify them thusly;

1. Gold Standard (G.S.) – dissection

2. I std. removed from G.S. – DEXA Scan

3. II std. removed from G.S. – Bioelectrical Impedance Analysis (BIA), Body Plethysmography (Bod Pod), Fat Calipers

4. III std. removed from G.S. – Whole body water displacement

As the number in the list gets higher, the amount of mathematical gymnastics increases factorially. This means that there are assumptions built into the black box, projected numbers which unilaterally alter the KPI that your machine spits out for things like body fat percentage. So yes, this means that DEXA has assumptions built into it which make it inaccurate – to some extent. You may be surprised that calipers and BIA are on the same level of accuracy. The reason here is they use the same mathematical equation used to calculate compositions. The BIA device uses hydration as a medium to obtain density information, then feeds it into a similar equation to the one used by caliper-based collection systems. The only difference here, is that a computer is "pinching" you, not a moody, emotional human. The same goes for BodPod. If you move at all, even a finger twitch, you will distort the collection of the computer's "pinch". This throws a monkey wrench into the software and produces an inaccurate reading. You may be asking, "why not just use the mirror test?" Pretty damn good question, actually.

I use a BIA scanner for my body comp tests. I use an 8-sensor hand-and-foot measuring device which is the second to the highest electrical power available on the market. This produces the highest possible BIA accuracy. I control for hydration by giving 2 days' notice to the athletes, no alcohol, 2 liters of water per day, and no workouts 6 hours before testing. Even with all this, the variability in body fat is over 1% between tests and over 1kg. of lean mass between tests. This is important because a shift of 1% upward may not mean any change at all. As I said before, I inform my thresholds based on my intimate knowledge of the machine and how it measures the athlete. The reason I pick BIA over calipers is that I can test an athlete in 30 seconds and get all my data, which is logged for me and ready to print. I can test an entire team in 20 minutes, impossible with calipers. As I have said before, data should make us fast – not slow the team down.

EVALUATE TRANSFER

I hope that these past pages have given you some inspiration. The things we discussed are not ground-breaking science, but the process of how to create it. Transfer is a process of shaking your assumptions about what the state of sports form means for your team. Pulling these assumptions up by the roots and dissecting them for inconsistencies. Technology can help here, especially with the right mindset. Once you have a fully formed structure in place you can begin the process of transfer. Remember the foundational principles:

1. Perspective – test what you can communicate

2. Commitment – test with integrity

3. Agility – test for application

In team sport, you can't train for transfer by yourself. You will need the entire coaching team (all of the tactical members) in order to achieve it. I hope that you will consider this, and the principles outlined in this chapter as you pursue it. I will close this essay with a quote from the Godfather of Transfer, Dr. Anatoliy Pavlovich Bondarchuk;

"A good coach tests all the time."

Who is Jake Jensen?

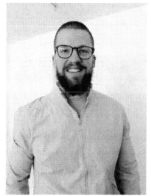

Jake is the Head Strength and Conditioning Coach for the Eisbaeren Berlin Hockey Club, in Berlin Germany.

He is primarily responsible for day-to-day training of the professional team and in addition directs S&C for the academy athletes of the U20 team, as well as consulting with the farm team club, the Lausitzer Fuchse. A native of Salt Lake City Utah, he completed his Undergraduate Degree at the University of Utah and his Master's Degree at Southern New Hampshire University. Fluent in four languages, Jake is a freelance Russian translator and interpreter having completed 5 books and several live events. He is also active in the academic community, publishing research with fellows at Humboldt University, Berlin. He currently lives in Berlin, Germany with his wife Brooke and their three sons.

7

Introduction to Force Plate Use and Neuromuscular Profiling

Karim Derqaoui

Force plate testing has long been the gold standard to analyze specific aspects of human performance such as the countermovement jump (CMJ). Within the laboratory setting, researchers aim to better understand the effects of training and other interventions on performance, how specific injuries affect movement potential, and gain further insight into the biomechanic signatures of various populations. In the rehabilitation setting, medical professionals utilize force plates during intake assessments for future comparisons, thus ensuring treatment interventions are effective and progress follows a given timeline. Finally, in the performance setting, a force plate system can establish a comprehensive profile and offer fast, reliable monitoring. This allows practitioners to create then adjust training and return to play protocols to maximize performance as well as reduce injury risk. Before diving into some force plate details, there are a few points that should be introduced first.

Force Plate Basics

A force plate is simply a traditional weighing scale, however a very sophisticated one that records force values over time. A bilateral force plate system has two plates, one for each leg or arm that is being tested during a bilateral test. This is the only configuration that can determine asymmetries during bilateral tests such a CMJ or a push up. Testing with a single plate will combine outputs from the left and right sides, making it impossible to determine the contributions from either during a movement. A robust resolution is considered to be 1000 Hz, in other words the software records 1000 data points per second to capture force-time data in great detail. With a bilateral force plate system collecting high-resolution data, biomechanical analyses can quantify several hundred key performance indicators from a single test like the CMJ. In order to understand where results (or *metrics*) come from, it's important to remember that force plates only measure force and time. Metrics should always be based on sound physics principles and calculations, not manipulated by proprietary algorithms that uses undisclosed equations. Although some force plate concepts need to be learned in the beginning, understanding of the process and knowledge of results will significantly empower professionals rather than partly removing them from the process in lieu of a "final athlete score" and an automatically generated exercise plan.

Neuromuscular profiling creates a framework for interpreting performance results and is founded on two central concepts. At any given time, an athlete possesses a unique set of physical traits that underpin **physical capacity** (hardware) and utilizes a cumulative **movement strategy** (software) to best achieve the given objective (*Image 1*). Sometimes the test requires an athlete to jump as high as they can or produce as much isometric force as possible. Other tests still simply require the athlete to land and hold a position. Whereas modifiable physical features can be semi-permanent, such as limb length and skeletal restrictions on joint effective range[1], some characteristics can be more easily modified through training and can yield favorable improvements in performance. Below are a few examples of such characteristics:

1. *Force generation capacity*: increased through individualized training programs that can improve eccentric (ECC) and/or concentric (CON) force output

2. *Muscle fiber distribution*: can change to various degrees to better meet intensity requirements of specific athletic endeavors (i.e.: repeat force production and/or rate of force development)

3. *Overall movement speed*: enhanced through rapid recruitment of larger, more powerful motor units (i.e.: increased efficiency between the descending pathway and muscle fibers)

4. *Body composition balance*: maximizes the ratio of force generating mass to non-essential mass (i.e.: lean body weight: excess adipose weight)

5. *Flexibility*: joint flexibility is desirable for greater range of motion while tendon stiffness should be increased to improve energy storage and transfer between movement phases

---

[1] Physical maturation during adolescence and the effects of age are two examples of changes that naturally occur over time but are not considered easily and/or voluntarily modifiable.

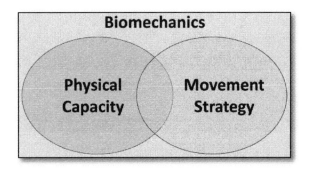

Image 1.

These physical characteristics determine an athlete's performance ceiling at any given time. However, huge variations exist among and between athletes in how they perform complex tasks such as jumping. Movement strategy describes the neuromuscular and compensatory methods an athlete utilizes to perform a given task. The movement strategy is much like a *signature* in that it's unique to each individual and naturally fluctuates to some degree between repetitions. Listed below are a few examples of what can influence a movement strategy during or between testing sessions:

1) Asymmetries from learned movement patterns or other factors (discussed later)

2) Unique physical attributes such as body mass, limb length, and joint ranges of motion

3) Fatigue compensation strategies

4) Adaptations that occur over time from training programs

Holistic interventions that improve both physical and movement qualities are often the most effective during performance training and rehabilitation. However, careful consideration should be given to what tests and metrics are selected prior to initial program creation.

Initial Assessment Overview: Test and Metric Selection

Force plates are extremely versatile and, when implemented correctly, offer a great deal of information on an athlete's specific physical attributes, movement strategy, and readiness status. The first ever assessment will always serve as an *athletic profile* or *baseline*. Initial data informs practitioners of what areas are deficient; monitoring then allows valid determination of progress and evaluation of program efficacy. Without an assessment, any performance or rehabilitation program would simply be guessing as to what the athlete needs in order to improve.

Test Selection

A concerted effort should always be made to select the most relevant tests for the given objective(s) in the present context. A simple hierarchy like this on can guide the process:

1) **Assessment rationale**: why are we testing (e.g.: baseline/intake, ongoing monitoring)?

2) **Participant status**: what is the readiness status of the individual (i.e.: maximum effort performance or restricted effort rehabilitation)?

3) **Test selection**: what performance qualities do we want to examine (e.g.: maximum strength, landing symmetry)?

4) **Metric selection**: what specific results will be most informative for these qualities (depends on test selection)?

Test selection should rely upon the underpinning rationale for assessment, overall performance goals, and what metrics are best placed to evaluate key attributes. Asking these questions will guide a practitioner to the right test(s) for a given context. Consider this possible scenario involving a colligate performance coach: the staff want to perform initial testing on the women's soccer team after their extended winter hiatus from structured training to know what condition they're in and where to focus their individual programs. Details from this example might resemble the following:

1. *Assessment rationale*: the players have had a non-supervised, 3-month off-season and the coach wants to know what condition they're returning in to mold appropriate training plans for each.

2. *Participant status*: 22/26 players are returning without any issues (maximum effort testing is not an issue) whereas 4/26 have various injuries (low(er) intensity assessments when needed).

3. *Test selection*: power is a key performance indicator in soccer and building strength is a spring-season priority for injury risk reduction during the competitive season; we can use force plates to test the CMJ and maximum strength output. With a good bilateral system and software, both tests offer asymmetry results and significant insights into injury risk potential.

4. *Metric selection*: the CMJ and Isometric tests on ForceDecks™ offer several dozen performance and movement strategy metrics.

Whereas most players can participate fully in all testing, those with injuries should be given special consideration. Sub-maximal effort tests can be used to establish neuromuscular capacity; prioritizing movement strategy and asymmetries over performance results from intense, high-impact tests is the most appropriate approach. For example, single leg balance and stability or landing technique assessment from various drop heights would be effective test options in Phase 2 of (most standard) ACL rehabilitation programs. In another example, an athlete returning from a calf strain may be able to perform isometric as well as land and hold tests from flat ground[2], but a CMJ or repeat hop test would be ill-advised in the early rehabilitation process. Most tests can be regressed to fit numerous scenarios; however, a good understanding of biomechanics is recommended to ensure valid results. Since each test involves a unique movement pattern and neuromuscular strategies, a practitioner can choose the best test to evaluate specific qualities. Although some tests directly evaluate primary sporting actions (e.g.: the CMJ for basketball and volleyball players), all athletes rely on expressing numerous qualities in a myriad of movement patterns beyond what a single test can determine. A practitioner should evaluate the underlying strength, power, and work:rest requirements of a sport or event. Afterwards they should determine the performance aptitudes required and, only then, select comprehensive testing options that fit best.

---

[2] Jumping from the opposite leg to the involved side requires no plantarflexion to initiate the jump; plantarflexion load will also be reduced if the forefoot delays contact with the plate until after initial impact.

Metric Selection

Selecting metrics for each assessment is a critical part of data analysis. The CMJ is an excellent example of a highly versatile and easily administered test that can be used in numerous contexts. Where athletic profiling is generally concerned, some metrics worth examining are ECC loading variables, peak power during the takeoff phase, landing results, and key asymmetry trends. Fatigue monitoring using the CMJ may include metrics that are more sensitive to neuromuscular changes. It is entirely possible to achieve an identical vertical jump height in a fatigued state by using an extended, less explosive movement strategy. Metrics for this type of fatigue monitoring may include squat depth, ECC duration, and peak force output. Finally, the CMJ can be an effective way to track rehabilitation progress and return to play. It would be worth examining ECC loading rates and peak values, whether using bilateral or unilateral tests. Improving limb coordination and maximum force output may greatly reduce injury and reinjury risks. Since an injury will almost always occur when tissue demand exceeds tissue capacity, whether it's acute or a chronic overload, it would be wise to raise the ceiling of an individual's capacity to give them sufficient reserves to safely meet demands.

The ECC loading phases can explain a great deal about movement strategy when the proper metrics are selected. The landing phase should be of particular interest since it involves potentially significant downward velocity and high force spikes which, when combined, require effective management for a safe touchdown. How the athlete performs reveals much about their injury risk as well as limb preference strategies. First, an athlete may have to absorb considerable forces above body mass when landing, depending on the drop height. **Peak landing force** will be greater after a longer flight time since velocity will be higher. Since an injury may have altered several components of landing coordination, a bilateral comparison is very useful to determine an athlete's ability to smoothly manage force-time requirements. In this case, **impulse results** can be used to determine force output over time and are an inclusive metric set to discover which side is performing deceleration work both ECC phases. Finally, the **rate of force development** during landing is much larger than during the preparation for the jump. Analysis may reveal if the athlete does not yet have the ability to load hard and fast on one side. These are three of the metrics that should be considered when analyzing the landing phase of any jump following an injury, but a closer examination will shed light on the details.

Hard and fast ECC loading, akin to what's produced during a landing, is common throughout infinite sport settings in both bilateral and unilateral contexts. From linear running to high-speed cutting maneuvers to Olympic weightlifting, rapid ECC loading is essential to maximize the stretch-shorten cycle, improve force production economy, and absorb force to redirect the body in another direction. The landing phase also requires increased neuromuscular coordination. After the athlete first contacts the ground, afferent signals report the rate and magnitude of ECC loading to help coordinate a smooth deceleration of the body during landing. Landing requires forces potentially far above body weight over a much shorter time. When landing from a jump, the athlete will have achieved a specific downward velocity based on jump height that will need to be quickly decelerated to zero through ECC loading, otherwise the athlete risks collapsing on the floor. In other words, the athlete is traveling downward at speed and either their ECC muscle action or the ground will get them to stop almost immediately after contact. This is in contrast to what occurs during ECC loading of the CMJ preparation phase. An athlete can choose to limit downward velocity and extend duration, resulting in relatively low force required over an unlimited amount of time to reach the bottom of the squat. The preparation for the CMJ begins in a static position with unlimited ground contact time, thus proprioceptive reflexes do not have to contend with fast force generation many times above body weight after a flight phase. Doing so will objectively determine how willing/able an athlete is to accept load on the injured limb.

Data Interpretation: Brief Review of Asymmetries

Asymmetry results can be very impactful in numerous contexts, informing practitioners on both performance and injury-risk status. Although there continues to be active discussions within the scientific and practitioner communities about how to classify asymmetry status, any apparent lack of consensus is generally accepted to be due to differences among individuals, groups, and relevant conditions that significantly impact test results. Therefore, asymmetry analysis should only ever be considered a risk indicator of injury, but never a *predictor*. Understanding asymmetry results in both healthy and injured athletes is critical; it establishes a framework of normative trends within a given cohort to which future evaluations can be compared. One significant strength of asymmetry analysis is that the measuring unit is universal and does not need to be analyzed relative to the participant. In nearly all circumstances, absolute values are reported as a percentage difference (%) between performance results during bilateral tests.[3] The challenge becomes knowing what level of difference is acceptable given relevant contextual factors, however knowledge and experience both play a role in that determination. For example, a 75% difference in a key metric is likely undesirable regardless of sport, position, or even injury history. Asymmetries may simply be a function of long-term participation in a particular sport or position. With that in mind, both average and maximum asymmetries should be taken into account during analysis. Practitioners should attempt to answer the following questions about results:

1. Does the athlete exhibit a compensatory movement strategy?

2. Is the asymmetry magnitude large enough to justify intervention?

3. Are there phase-specific asymmetries that warrant more attention?

4. Is there any history of injury that warrants more scrutiny?

5. Is there any variability or trends that would signal cause for greater or lesser concern?

6. It is reasonable to expect to see asymmetries for athletes from different sport backgrounds?

Analyzing asymmetries may seem to be a complicated process but understanding some key concepts will help create a straightforward, flexible system. We will now examine six considerations for asymmetry analysis.

---

[3] Or unilateral compared to each other.

Asymmetry Magnitude

Magnitude simply refers to the absolute size of an asymmetry, without consideration for the direction (i.e.: left or right). A 0% asymmetry for a given metric would suggest an individual does not favor one limb over the other (during that specific repetition). However, if the magnitude of an asymmetry is greater than 0%, the implications are not as clear. A typical asymmetry for a single group is unlikely to be indicative of all populations, therefore results must be interpreted with caution. It could be argued that highly specialized athletes in very homogenous groups (e.g.: Major League Baseball (MLB) pitchers, fencers) have an elevated propensity for large asymmetry values. A descending distribution curve for a specific sub-category would therefore be skewed right compared to the population (i.e.: higher asymmetries in more of the sample than the population). Whether a group has high variation or not, a rating system can be created by simply collecting data and observing asymmetry trends within a sub-group.

Change in Asymmetry Magnitude

Changes in asymmetry may be influenced by both acute fatigue as well as ongoing training adaptations. For an example of acute changes, consider an athlete who averages 9% asymmetry for a given metric 48 hours before competition. The same athlete averages 25% asymmetry for the same metric *the day after* competition. This might suggest that, when in a fatigued state, the asymmetry is magnified and could suggest the athlete overly relied on one side during competition (localized fatigue) and/or central changes amplify the movement strategy imbalance (nervous system fatigue). Variations in magnitude over time can help identify improvements or warn practitioners of a developing problem. If an athlete displays a 5% asymmetry on the first day of preseason testing but that difference grows each week, this may indicate an issue is developing. Conversely, if a client recovering from ACL reconstruction begins their rehabilitation at 40% asymmetry, but consistently reduces this asymmetry over time, this may indicate positive progress. These changes are often not perceived by the athlete, let alone quantified to any reliable degree. Using dual force plate measurement can identify changes in magnitude and interventions can happen earlier than would otherwise be possible with subjective analysis only.

Influence of Previous Injury on Asymmetry

Immediately following an injury, force production capacity and movement mechanics will be altered in accordance with injury severity (i.e.: acute responses). However, the resultant state may go on to affect an athlete long term (i.e.: chronic adaptations). Depending on the nature of the injury and subsequent rehabilitation process, there may be limits as to the amount of improvement possible for an asymmetry. Examples of this are commonly observed following injuries such as an ACL tear or after procedures when surgical implants are required. In such scenarios it becomes a question of management, both of expectations and training programs. An asymmetry analysis should consider how previous setbacks may still affect the athlete and how that may change the goals of their exercise program.

Sport/Position

Asymmetries can develop naturally in response to repetitive actions but may not necessarily be cause for concern. For example, an MLB pitcher may have the most asymmetrical physical demands of any athlete in elite sport, considering each of his limbs has drastically different skill and power demands.[4] In other sporting contexts, elite road cyclists and power lifters could be among the most symmetrical since their force and power demands are evenly distributed in bilateral fashion. While a pitcher may show substantial asymmetries between their pitching and glove hand and between their drive and land leg, this does not necessarily mean that they are at any elevated risk of injury. If a pitcher is generally healthy, performing at a competitive level, and their magnitudes of asymmetry do not fluctuate greatly over time, a relatively high

---

[4] This asymmetry is further compounded by the fact MLB pitchers need to 1) produce as much force as possible from their glove hand and drive leg, 2) that there is little/no variation on the movement patterns they employ, 3) there is no limit to how many hitters a pitcher can face per inning, and 4) games can continue indefinitely because there is no timeclock and a winner must be declared in most instances. This combination of factors ensures pitchers throw at the very highest intensity possible for pretty much as long as they possibly can, ensuring high volumes each time they're on the mound.

asymmetry may be considered perfectly normal. The same can be the case for less obvious factors, such as subtle differences in anthropometry, physiology, or other factors, again alluding to comparing intra-personal to wider population norms.

Consistency of Inter-Phase Asymmetries

Asymmetries can occur with any given metric, whether it's a singular point (e.g.: peak takeoff force), a value of force over time (e.g.: ECC braking impulse), or a rate of force applied (e.g.: ECC deceleration rate of force development). To thoroughly understand asymmetries, it is important to analyze an entire movement, looking for similarities and differences across phases and/or landmarks. For example, consider the three major phases of the CMJ test: 1) ECC, 2) CON, and 3) Landing. Individuals may exhibit minimal asymmetry in one phase while showing significant asymmetry in another phase. Such a phenomenon may be explained by a number of different factors. For example, an athlete may be subconsciously "protecting" one limb from rapid loading (e.g.: RFD and impulse metrics) and/or heavy loading (e.g.: higher average force or impulse asymmetries). In either case, the specific phase or variable in which asymmetries occur can provide significant insights as to why and how an athlete moves as they do.

Consistency of Inter-Trial Asymmetries

Performing several repetitions of a jump or other movement may yield asymmetry results of significantly different magnitudes and directions. Consider an athlete who performs five drop jump tests from the same height and registers a consistent asymmetry of 12% right-sided dominance across numerous metrics and phases (Figure 2). Although the magnitude may not be a cause for great concern, the fact the individual consistently stresses one limb more than the other may warrant investigation, or at least justify closer monitoring over time. Compare this to another athlete who performs the same test, however with a variety of asymmetry magnitudes from 2% - 40% which randomly alternate between left- and right-dominance across all metrics (Figure 3). Although peak asymmetry magnitudes appear higher in some of the trials, average asymmetry across the entire testing session (i.e.: inclusive of both left and right sides) may be closer to 0%. This large variance may be completely normal, resulting from different movement strategies from trial to trial. This might also suggest the athlete is comfortable in accepting load and producing force on both limbs equally and can solve a variety of "movement equations." While such results seem highly variable, this athlete's performance profile might actually be protective and indicate they may be well-prepared to tolerate variable loading on both limbs.

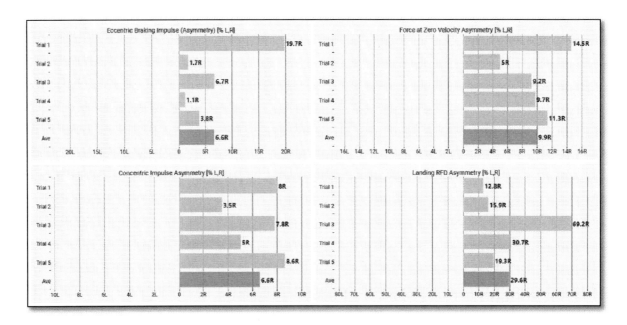

Figure 2.

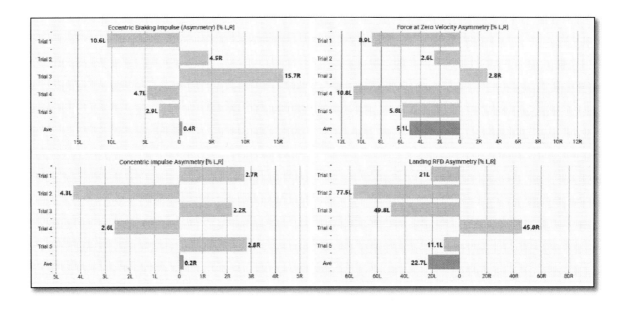

Figure 3.

Closing Remarks

Force plates are an incredibly reliable and highly sophisticated assessment tool that supports numerous performance and rehabilitation contexts. With the right setup, testing is very efficient and practitioners can gain access to an abundance of data. Minimal training is required for the acquisition and interpretation of metrics such as a jump height, relative power, and asymmetry results. However, some systems offer dozens of tests and hundreds of metrics, giving an organization immediate flexibility and room to build upward as staff experience grows. Following a sound rationale for test and metric selection is the best means to ensure maximum validity for all assessments. However, correlations can appear in unexpected ways amidst data sets so experimentation with force plate tests and metrics is highly encouraged.

REFERENCES

1. Cohen, D, et al. Single Vs Double Leg Countermovement Jump Tests. Aspetar 34–41 (N.D.).

2. Cormack, SJ, et al. Neuromuscular And Endocrine Responses Of Elite Players During An Australian Rules Football Season. Int'l J Of Sports Physiology And Performance 3, 439–453 (2008).

3. Gathercole, RJ, et al. Effect Of Acute Fatigue And Training Adaptation On Countermovement Jump Performance In Elite Snowboard Cross Athletes. J Strength Cond Res 29, 37–46 (2015).

4. Gathercole, RJ, et al. Alternative Countermovement-Jump Analysis To Quantify Acute Neuromuscular Fatigue. Int'l J Of Sports Physiology And Performance 10, 84–92 (2015).

5. Hart, LM, et al. Previous Injury Is Associated With Heightened Countermovement Jump Force-Time Asymmetries In Professional Soccer Players. Trans. Sports Medicine 2, 256–262 (2019).

6. Jordan, MJ, et al. Asymmetry And Thigh Muscle Coactivity In Fatigued Anterior Cruciate Ligament–Reconstructed Elite Skiers. Medicine Sci Sports Exerc 49, 11–20 (2017).

7. Knezevic, OM, et al. Asymmetries In Explosive Strength Following Anterior Cruciate Ligament Reconstruction. Knee 21, 1039–1045 (2014).

8. Stone, MH, et al. Using The Isometric Mid- Thigh Pull In The Monitoring Of Weightlifters: 25+ Years Of Experience. Professional Strength And Conditioning (2019).

9. Turner, AN, et al. Total Score Of Athleticism: Holistic Athlete Profiling To Enhance Decision-Making. Strength Cond J 41, 91–101 (2019).

10. Whitmer, TD, et al. Accuracy Of A Vertical Jump Contact Mat For Determining Jump Height And Flight Time. J Of Applied Sport Science Research 29, 877–881 (2015).

11. Wing, C, et al. Monitoring Athlete Load: Data Collection Methods And Practical Recommendations. Strength Cond J 40, 1 (2018).

Who is Karim Derqaoui?

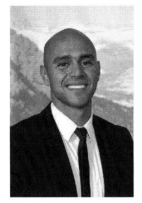

Karim Derqaoui is in his third year with VALD Performance. He oversees numerous global educational initiatives across many of the company's systems, however largely regarding ForceDecks. His background is centered on performance training, sport science, and end-stage rehab in elite athletics. His experience includes training Major League Soccer teams, D1 college athletics, and international consulting. He has advanced degrees in Sport Science and Exercise Physiology, as well as post-graduate research and teaching in neurophysiology. Originally from Morocco, Karim was raised in France and San Francisco but now calls New Jersey his home.

8

Navigating the Rehab Process

Terrence "TK" Kennell

Synopsis:

Developing and integrating criteria-based rehabilitation that is holistic in nature and breaks down the various stages or the process. Using objectivity to as our guide throughout; to help take much of the guess work out of it and stack the deck in our favour.

The Return to Performance (RTP) process has historically been that somewhat messy middle ground within our profession where roles and responsibilities between the performance and medical staff can become a bit unclear and communication break downs can lead to the hinderance of an athlete's progression to full performance. Commonly medical staffs, be it team doctor, physical therapist, or athletic trainer, will have somewhat of a general timeline for various injuries. These timelines of course function merely as a reference guide, and are in no way prescriptive, as injuries are case by case and multi-factorial. These timeline references can be used in the early RTP stages, in the initial meetings between performance and medical staff to determine what some of the agreed upon criteria/benchmarks are that need to be accomplished before progressing the athlete forward in the process and, therefore, helping plan out the early stages of RTP and clarifying all roles and responsibilities.

I will try and shed some light on my principles for the RTP process, and the objective measurements used in lower body injury RTP in this chapter. This will focus solely on the lower body due my past experience showing that the upper body can be a little trickier, but I have a few ideas I have stolen from much smarter people. This all begins by working backwards from the game demands of the athlete. This is what guides not only our physical preparation, but also the technical and tactical reintegration process. Hopefully in doing so we are not throwing the athlete straight into the fire that can be the chaos of sport without exposing them to the demands of the game in an isolated, more controlled setting, and then slowly layering in more stress and chaos. When dealing with a longer term RTP like an ACL repair, this is especially important. I also want to try and layout my past experiences on how to define clearer roles and responsibilities in RTP between the performance and medical staff so that the two are always working together for the common goal of making the athlete better. Although looked at as a chance to get healthy, RTP is also a chance for the injured player to become a better athlete.

Creating & Defining stages in RTP

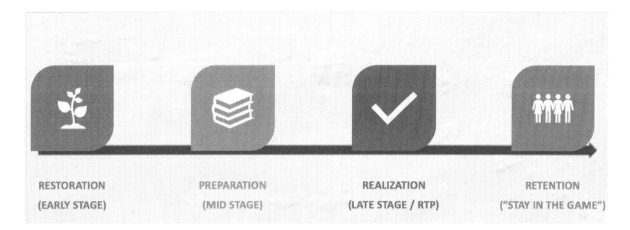

The stages or phases of RTP allow for the ability to create common language in communication between staff, as well as player. These stages provide insight into what goals and benchmarks are along the path and who takes the lead in that stage. I've worked with the general concept of a 60:40 split with regards to who takes the lead and who the athlete is spending the most time with during a certain stage of RTP. We will break down each stage in a bit more detail as well as to the adaptation being trained in that stage.

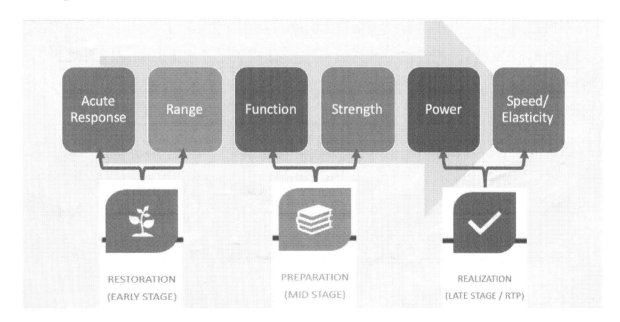

Restoration/Early stage: This is that immediate post injury stage, heavily led by the medical staff dealing with acute response to the new trauma along with wound care, reduction of swelling, inflammatory responses, etc. Generally, many things are out of the scope of practice for the performance staff. In this stage things that we, as performance practitioners, can/should do is work alongside our medical staff and find out what the athlete can do. There is usually three other limbs and a trunk that can all be trained in some capacity, so work to prevent detraining of the rest of the body as much as you can. The main adaptations were looking for in this restoration stage are acute response and range of motion to help prepare the tissues for load down the line. This stage is vital, as it sets the foundation for the rest of the RTP process. General goals of this stage are to: alleviate pain relative to injury, normal active and passive range of motion, and treat any contributing postural dysfunction. In figure 1 you will see some of the measurements that have been used to aid in objectifying this restoration stage. As stated earlier, this stage is the time where the staffs can meet and devise a plan of attack going forward, identify KPIs, plan for what you already know, come up with possibilities for the "Plan B's" that will be needed at some point, and review athletes' previous data if applicable.

Preparation/Mid Stage: The second stage of the RTP/Rehab Process tends to be the longest. We are looking to restore full "normal" joint function of the injured area while also beginning to increase the load on the healing tissue. The adaptation emphasis of this stage is function and strength. The roles and responsibilities of the practitioners involved can begin to lean more heavily to the S&C coach taking the lead, a simple breakdown would just be roughly a 60:40 split in terms of the athlete spending the bulk of their time with the S&C coach in terms of progressive overloading and moving forward in the process.

When looking at improving function of the injured limb, we are looking to encourage multi-planar movement competency at low intensities while remaining relatively pain free, or quite low on the pain scale depending on the injury. The goal to increase neuromuscular input to the affected structure(s) while utilizing appropriate load management with regards to reps/sets/intensities. The simple progression of increasing very low-level work capacity prior to increasing frequency and intensity of load on those structures has shown success. The low-level work capacity helps in stacking the deck in our favor, so that the athlete can move in and out of foundational positions and can handle higher volume/low intensity work without significant fatigue or acute mal-responses. This time is also used as a chance to improve kinesthetic awareness in static and dynamic task using various closed and open chain movements.

The next adaptation we are chasing in this Preparation/Mid stage is strength. Naturally that's a fun one for strength & conditioning practitioners. The goal is to progressively overload the body to create neural and structural adaptations. Strength is generally our foundation of higher rates of force production and system robustness. We cannot optimize a system that is not robust initially as that can be a variable for re-injury in the future. Therefore, progressively looking to recruit higher motor units for enhancing maximal force outputs should be done before we progress to more ballistic and elastic training modalities. We are looking for hypertrophy adaptations in this stage as well to counteract any muscle atrophy lost post-surgery or from immobilization of a limb. Breadth and girth measurements serve as a great assessment to make sure we are getting any hypertrophic adaptations we are seeking during this stage. Baseline assessments are highly valuable and can help give us some general landmarks that we need to hit, or be at least within 10% of. If you have those for strength as well that's a huge benefit. The traditional weight room tests are always helpful to assess where an athlete is in terms of strength, looking at things like 3RMs, 2RMs, bar velocity at a certain percentage etc. are all valuable assessments to run for the exercises that are more pertinent to the program you run. If you are lucky enough to have a set of bilateral force plates, then there are some assessments I have found useful. For the lower body: SL ISO Squat, SL Peak Plantar Force, and isometric mid-thigh pull are my preferred evaluations. A key for these assessments, like any other evaluation, is that they should be done regularly so that you can properly track progress throughout the rehab process. The upper body assessment that has been found most useful is the Ash Test ITY. There are a few other upper body assessments on the force plates have that I have been toying around with, but I don't have enough experience with them to be confident with. These are the Davis's test, kneeling push up position land and hold (think altitude drop for push up). If you choose to play around with these upper body ones and find some success, please let me know.

The figure below shows a table of some of the assessments that would be used as various stages:

	Acute	Range	Function	Strength	Power	Speed/Elasticity
Ankle/Shin/Calf	Gait Assessment	Ankle DF Clearing Exam	Y Balance Test	SL Peak Plantar Force	CMJ and SL CMJ	DJ RSI 35cm SL DJ RSI 20cm 10-5 Hop Test
Knee	Girth Measurements	Flexion Extension	Y Balance Test	SL Iso Squat	CMJ and SL CMJ	DJ RSI 35cm SL DJ RSI 20cm
Hamstring	Palpable Tenderness	PSLR > 70 Deg	ASLR	Nordic Curl	Supine 90/90 RFD	N/A
Hip/Groin	N/A	N/A	Eccentric Step Down	ABD/ADD Force Frame	N/A	N/A
Trunk/Spine (?)	N/A	N/A	McGill trunk capacity/Extens or (Sorenson) Endurance Test	Isometric Trunk	N/A	N/A
Shoulder	N/A	N/A	Scapular Dyskinesis Test Davis Test	IR/ER force frame	ASH test RFD	Bench Press Throw Landmine Throw

Figure 1

Realization/ Late Stage: In this stage the foundations laid earlier are built upon as the athlete is getting closer to returning to sporting activity. The main goals are adaptations of power and speed/elasticity at this point in the RTP process. We are looking for force production at much higher rates of speed, so those adaptations take priority in the program. Moving forward in the progression of training means from extensive to intensive with ballistic exercises (throws) and stretch shortening cycle muscle/tendon interactions (jumps). In the weight room we can objectively gather some information to help us ensure the athlete is ready for the intensive means by using assessments like the 10-5 hop test and drop jumps to evaluate ground contact time, reactive strength index (RSI), and limb asymmetries, if we have a bilateral force plate. If force plates are not available, an adequate back up plan is to look at RSI and ground contact times using tools like a Just Jump Mat or a G-Flight. Throughout this phase the goal is to attempt to ensure that we are getting closer to higher CNS demands that are seen in sport. For a lower body injury, the athlete needs to be prepared for the massive ground reaction forces of sprinting as much as possible. If it's an upper body injury, then we are trying to prepare the body for throwing, tackling, absorbing contact and/or whatever the sport demands.

The figure below provides insight into the types of forces were trying to prepare body for when it comes to sprinting:

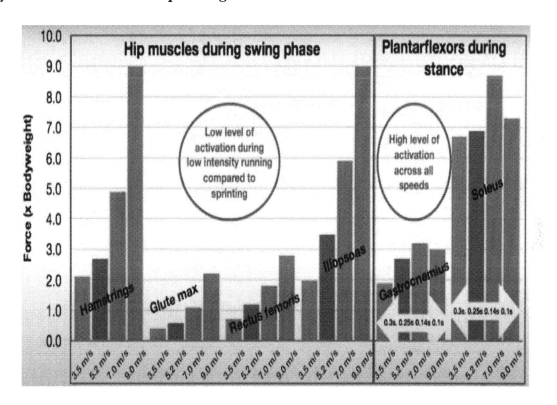

The late stage is also where the field or court is taking more of a priority over training in the weight room. The athlete is being exposed to not only a higher amount of ground contacts with jumps/plyometrics, but we also have marches (can be done in mid stage usually), skips, bounds, decelerations, non-resisted and resisted running, shuffles, cuts, curves, etc. It's a constant progression of layering stimulus/stress and seeing how the athlete responds. The continuum I use as a framework for how I progress on field work is Tom Farrow's Skill-Drill-Chaos. This progression functions as a simple way to see how you build your sessions and determine the athlete's re-integration into practice. The progression starts with pre-determined closed skill work to higher speed/force drills, and eventually into reactive chaotic environments that are required by the sport. Matt Taberner's "Control-Chaos Continuum" paper also lays out a great framework for progressing on field rehab along with practice re-integration and is something I use as a reference whenever needed.

HIGH CONTROL

SESSIONS	<8 GAME LOAD**
TYPE	RETURN TO RUNNING PHASE 1 (RTR1)
CONDITIONING EMPHASIS	THRESHOLD ENDURANCE (80-85% MAX*) INTENSIVE ENDURANCE (70-80% MAX*)
DESCRIPTION	LINEAR RUNNING (> FROM ALTER-G - 90% BW) LOW MAGNITUDE ACC/DEC LOW VOLUME EXPLOSIVE DISTANCE LOW MUSCULOSKELETAL IMPACT FORCES END OF STAGE INTRODUCTION TO HSR (INJURY SPECIFIC) EXAMPLES: 3X5, 4X6 (1-4XMINS) EXAMPLE: 3X3, 4X4 (1-2XMINS PB)
LOAD EMPHASIS (INJURY SPECIFIC)	>ACC / TD; <DEC / <EXPO/ <HSR
NO. OF SESSIONS	2-4

MODERATE CONTROL

SESSIONS	<8.35-0.45 GAME LOAD**
TYPE	RETURN TO RUNNING: CONTROLLED CHANGE OF DIRECTION PHASE 2 (RTR2)
CONDITIONING EMPHASIS	THRESHOLD ENDURANCE (80-85% MAX*) INTENSIVE ENDURANCE (70-80% MAX*)
DESCRIPTION	INTRODUCE COD WITH/WITHOUT BALL (45-180° TURNING) >LINEAR RUNNING SPEEDS (FARTLEK) >MUSCULOSKELETAL IMPACT FORCES/JOINT DEMANDS INTRO SHORT-RANGE TECHNICAL E.G. PASSING EXAMPLE: 3-5X3-4XMINS (1-2XMINS PB)
LOAD EMPHASIS (INJURY SPECIFIC)	>ACC / TD; >DEC / >HSR /<EXPO
NO. OF SESSIONS	3-4

CONTROL>CHAOS

SESSIONS	<0.40-0.60 GAME LOAD**
TYPE	INTENSIVE / EXTENSIVE
CONDITIONING EMPHASIS	EXTENSIVE TEMPO DEVELOPMENT LEVEL 1 (<75-70% MS) V̇O₂MAX DEVELOPMENT (>85% MAX*) THRESHOLD ENDURANCE (80-85% MAX*) INTENSIVE ENDURANCE (70-80% MAX*)
DESCRIPTION	COD WITH*/WITHOUT BALL (ALL TURNS) RUNNING SPEEDS (>60-70% MS - HSR) (FARTLEK) LOW VOLUME/INTENSITY P+M/P/OP >MUSCULOSKELETAL IMPACT FORCES/JOINT DEMANDS >ACC/DEC PREPARATION PROGRESSION OF TECHNICAL SKILLS INTENSIVE: 4-6X1-2XMINS (1-2XMINS PB) EXTENSIVE: 4-6X4-6XMINS (2-3XMINS PB) TEMPO/AEROBIC POWER INTERVAL RUNNING (17-34) (45-195)
LOAD EMPHASIS (INJURY SPECIFIC)	>ACC / TD; >DEC / >HSR / >EXPO; >ACC / TD; >DEC / >HSR / >EXPO (MS)
NO. OF SESSIONS	3-4

MODERATE CHAOS

SESSIONS	*0.55-0.70 GAME LOAD**
TYPE	INTENSIVE / EXTENSIVE
CONDITIONING EMPHASIS	EXTENSIVE TEMPO LEVEL 1 (<75-70% MS) V̇O₂MAX DEVELOPMENT (>85% MAX*) THRESHOLD ENDURANCE (80-85% MAX*) INTENSIVE ENDURANCE (70-80% MAX*)
DESCRIPTION	>RUNNING SPEEDS *(>75% MS) >HSR ACCUMULATED SPRINT EXPOSURE POSITIONAL P+M/P/OP >ACC/DEC DEMANDS (POSITIONAL) >MUSCULOSKELETAL IMPACT/JOINT DEMANDS VOLUME/INTENSITY (INCLUDING TECHNICAL SKILLS) SPEED:3-10S (1.5-1:10) SPEED ENDURANCE PRODUCTION/MAINTENANCE INTENSIVE: 20-45S/1-3MIN (1-3MINS PB) EXTENSIVE: 6-8MINS (2-3MINS PB)
LOAD EMPHASIS (INJURY SPECIFIC)	>ACC / TD; >DEC / >HSR />EXPO; >ACC / TD; >DEC / >HSR /<EXPO (MS)
NO. OF SESSIONS	3-5 (DEPENDANT UPON TRAINING METHOD)

HIGH CHAOS

SESSIONS	<70 GAME LOAD**
TYPE	INTENSIVE / EXTENSIVE
CONDITIONING EMPHASIS	SPEED (>85% MS) EXTENSIVE TEMPO LEVEL 2 (<85-75% MS) V̇O₂MAX DEVELOPMENT (>85% MAX*) THRESHOLD ENDURANCE (80-85% MAX*) INTENSIVE ENDURANCE (70-80% MAX*)
DESCRIPTION	>RUNNING SPEEDS (>90% MS) >HSR/SPR ACCUMULATED RTT POSITIONAL SPECIFIC DEMANDS ACC/DEC DEMANDS (POSITIONAL) >MUSCULOSKELETAL IMPACT/JOINT DEMANDS >MATCH-DAY TYPE PREPARATION (POSITIONAL - TECHNICAL SKILLS) SPEED:3-10S (1.5-1:10) SPEED ENDURANCE PRODUCTION/MAINTENANCE INTENSIVE: 20-45S/1-3MIN (2-3MINS PB) EXTENSIVE: 4-8MINS (2-3MINS PB)
LOAD EMPHASIS (INJURY SPECIFIC)	>ACC / TD; >DEC / >HSR />EXPO; >ACC / TD; >DEC / >HSR />EXPO (MS)
NO. OF SESSIONS	3-5 (DEPENDANT UPON TRAINING METHOD)

Figure from "Control to Chaos continuum"

Retention: When an athlete fully exits the rehab process, the goal is to never have to work with them in that context again. Having a plan for the athlete as they start training fully with the team and start playing games is highly valuable so to essentially stay on top of anything that may come up. Having 1-2 assessments that you can have the athlete do regularly throughout the year is very beneficial to track progress and try to get ahead of any potential mal responses that come up from returning to full participation.

The rehab process should always be viewed as a time for the athlete to get better as a whole. It's more than simply coming back healthy, that's the bare minimum! It's about coming back ready to perform at a high level. Having criteria and objectively based progressions is beneficial to determine how to advance an athlete forward and help discern what underlying issues can be addressed as well. That may have a long-term positive impact on the athlete's success.

Thank you very much for reading this far,

Thank you, Jay, for inviting me to do this! Really appreciate it.

REFERENCES

1. Matt Taberner: "Control to Chaos Continuum"

2. "Sports Injury prevention and rehabilitation" Edited by David Joyce and Daniel Lewindon

3. Bill Knowles: "Reconditioning"

4. "Prescription of Training Load in relation to loading and unloading phases of training" – AIS

5. "Force Plate use in monitoring and testing" George Beckham

6. "Understanding the key phases of the Counter-Movement jump Force Time Curve" John J. McMahon

7. "Football Rehabilitation: How to safely reintegrate, avoid re-injury and prepare players for the demands of the premier league" Damian Roden

Who is Terrence "TK" Kennell, aka Young Terrence?

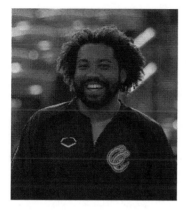

"TK" is the High-Performance Director Kansas City Women's Soccer NWSL, and formerly the S&C Rehab Coordinator for the Houston Astros. He served as S&C for rugby clubs in London and Japan, and also gained experience in pro mixed martial arts, boxing, tennis, and basketball. He has an undergraduate degree from Arkansas State and received a post-graduate degree in applied sports and exercise physiology from St. Mary's University in London. Born in Anchorage, AK, Kennell was raised in a U.S. Army family that moved extensively around the US and lived in a few countries as well.

9

Reevaluating Conditioning

Simple Strategies for Maximum Results

Jay DeMayo

The evolution of conditioning the athlete in strength and conditioning has been an intriguing cycle to observe. It's one that I have found myself being duped into some different areas of the spectrum of extreme "new" ideas, means, or methods that show up each year. I have not been immune to the 'fear of missing out" (FOMO) that comes from scrolling on Instagram or Twitter and seeing all these great things coaches are doing and how successful their athletes WILL become because of them. Going through this process for greater than fifteen years has brought about a great deal of experience, or better stated, experiments due to this FOMO. As my career has evolved, these different experiments have occurred, and my time with basketball has increased, I seem to come back to some methods that have, in our opinion, been the most successful when it comes to increasing these athletes conditioning. Prior to us diving into the "what, why, how" of this aspect of our program, there are some very important things we need to discuss that are unique to the world of basketball at this level. Each of these need to be accounted for and have had a major impact in our programming decisions. Also, please keep in mind that each situation is unique so what works for one may not work for another, but hopefully these next few pages will help open discussion and ideas to how we can all do better by our athletes.

When discussing things that need to be accounted for, when setting up the program, the first is one of those cringy slogans you've seen on a t-shirt or hashtag somewhere, *"basketball never stops"*. As disgusting as this statement is it's the complete truth. To give you an example of it, let's just look at this past season, even with COVID, and how it leads into next season (2021-22). Our team reported July 15th to begin their progression back to basketball activity. This, of course, was not full speed. In fact, the initial phases were quite controlled, and they progressed throughout the summer leading into practice. Once full practice started in September we didn't stop for more than 5 days in a row until the season ended on March 25th. There were off days once every seven days, or twice every fourteen days, as per NCAA rules, but there were no true extended breaks. After roughly two weeks of an extended break we began off season workouts again, this will last for about 2 weeks, and then the team will get three weeks off before returning for the summer. Once here, we would typically have eight weeks of countable athletic related activity (CARA) weeks in the summer, but because this is a "foreign trip" year, once those 8 weeks are finished we begin practice. We have

10 of those, so roughly 2 more weeks, and then would travel/play games elsewhere. Due to the pandemic the trip part may not happen, but we are looking at how we could keep it domestic so that we could still practice and play. These trips typically last 10 days to 2 weeks, and once we return home the players get one week "off" at the end of the summer prior to the start of classes. They would then return to campus in late August when we would start individual instruction and training, which will roll right into practice. Once we start practice we would roll straight through the season, ending (hopefully) in early April. So, once we look at this time, spanning 90 weeks, these young people will have, roughly, 7 or 8 weeks off. This occurs once a "career" in each players 4 years in college as well.

Why is this important? The fact that these athletes are participating in their sporting activity, or at the least in some form of practice and playing (pick-up), for a vast majority of the year SHOULD indicate that the need for specific preparation is being taken care of. This should make sense to all of us who love to discuss our role in building the robustness of the athlete by looking at the bioenergetic demands of the sport and training the athletes accordingly. If they're always practicing, playing in controlled environments (drills and small sided games like 4v4 or 2v2) then this box is ticked. For this reason, our vision has shifted to different buckets, but it's not the only reason why we have decided to do so.

This is also about building throughout the general physical preparation phase for the athletes. Now, I'm more than willing to sit and listen to people tell me how we will never have a GPP phase because, as stated above, basketball never stops. Due to that, we would appear to not have time to develop these general qualities because the athletes are never able to concentrate on their general training. There's a ton of different ways to describe this concept. You can't serve two masters. Can't ride two horses with one butt. Even though, up until very recently I would agree with you, I think that's an even greater reason to develop these general qualities. This is because they are always participating in some form of skill work and technical tactical training for their sport. So, with the respect to their general physical preparation, as we progressively increase loads in training (both volume and intensity) the athlete adapts (improves these qualities) in conjunction with working on (and hopefully improving) their skill. The thought process to this is simple, the more they practice while they're getting stronger and in better shape, the greater possibility for this to carry-over is to their sport. This also fits into the "bucket" idea mentioned above that many coaches discuss when referring to in season training. It's just going to last a lot longer with basketball because of how few the actual "down times" are. With all that in mind, we can "fill the buckets" that they aren't getting at practice to help increase the athlete's ability to be resilient to stress. This is, after all, what we say we do, right?

It is also imparative that we examine this time of the training calendar. We are in the General Physical Preparation Phase. In my mind, this is where we go to our bread and butter. At this time of year we focus on strength and conditioning. This is the time to build general strength in a progressive manner while building their general endurance qualities. This could also be stated as building the base of the pyramid that so many of us in the performance world reference constantly. But why build those two at this point of the year while the athletes are practicing. We have come to this conclusion due to the work of Dr. Issurin. In his book *"Block Periodization"*, these are two qualities that are compatible to train together. Now, I'm not sure if there is some sort of exercise Tinder or whatever where these compatibilities were found, but he's a pretty smart person who's looked into these things for a long time, so in this instance, I'm going to take his word for it. The second reason is that during a regular year (whatever that is) there is typically a 3-4-week break following the traditional weeks of CARA in the summer. So, while we have roughly two months to prepare the athletes, we then have about a month where they go home, and assumingly take a break from our training. There have been two different thought processes that I have heard coaches use to handle this time period. The first is to try to "over train" the athletes and allow them to "super compensate" when they go home. If I'm going to be completely frank, I'm not sure I believe this actually will occur in that amount of time for two reasons. First, that's more time then is actually needed for a realization phase to occur, unless they are truly over trained and breaking down. If they are at that point we may have greater issues. Secondly, we know that when they go home, most of these athletes are going to go work with their "guy". They may not be training the way we were when they were on campus, shoot they may not be doing any non-sport skill work at all, but they aren't taking the time "off" to rest either. If they're not, then they aren't completely recovering either. Disclaimer: something in my head just doesn't think trying to over train kids is a good idea, but that's just me. So that leads us to the second option and back to Dr. Vladimir Issurin and "*Block Periodization*".

Training Compatibility	
Dominant Training Modality	**Compatible Training Modalities**
Aerobic Endurance	Alactic sprint abilities, Strength endurance (Aerobic), Maximum strength, Hypertrophy
Glycolytic Endurance	Strength Endurance (anaerobic), Aerobic restoration, Aerobic-anaerobic (mixed) endurance
Alactic Sprints	Aerobic Endurance, Explosive strength, Maximum Strength, Hypertrophy, Aerobic restoration
Maximum Strength/ Hypertrophy	Maximum strength, flexibility, aerobic restoration
Learning new technical elements	Any kind of training modalities after the primary/dominant task

Adapted from: Issurin, V. (2008). "Block Periodization: Breakthrough in Sports Training." New York, NY: Ultimate Athlete Concepts.

Residual Training Effects		
Motor Ability	**Retention**	**Physiological**
Oxidative Energy System	30±5	Increased number of aerobic enzymes, mitochondria, capillary density, hemoglobin capacity, glycogen storage, higher rate of fat metabolism
Strength	30±5	Improvement of neural mechanism, muscle hypertrophy
Glycolytic Energy System	18±4	Increased anaerobic enzymes, buffering capacity and glycogen storage, higher possibility of lactate accumulation
Repeat-Power	15±5	Improved aerobic/ anaerobic enzymes, improved local blood circulation and lactate tolerance, repeat sprint ability
ATP/CR-P	5±3	Enhanced resynthesis of CR-P
Speed	5±3	Improved neuromuscular interactions and motor control, increases anaerobic power

Adapted from: Issurin, V. (2008), "Block Periodization: Breakthrough in Sports Training." New York, NY: Ultimate Athlete Concepts.

Both graphics from The Coach's Guide to Programming and Periodization: Residual Effects, Compatibility, and The Needs Analysis by Nicholas Bronkall Published by Elitefts.com at: https://www.elitefts.com/education/coaching-education/the-coachs-guide-to-programming-and-periodization-residual-effects-compatibility-and-the-needs-analysis/

Quick pause here, if you don't have this book go over to **https://uaconcepts.com** right now and order a copy because it's a must for your reference library.

Ok, back on track, Dr. Issurin shares with us that there are residual training effects to training each specific quality in an athlete. So not only has he shared with us what we can train together, but he's also informed us how long these qualities can "hold on" before they need to be trained again. You don't need to be a fan of the sensational 1990's classic by Wilson Phillips to understand how important residual training effects are in this situation. Holding onto these training effects for the month they're away is vital, but what "qualities" hold on the longest? I'm going to go out on a limb and say that you probably guessed that aerobic conditioning and strength not only go together like peanut butter and jelly but also last the test of time, having the longest residual training effects, around a month. So even when we go on our "foreign tour" and we can't train for a few weeks, we shouldn't "lose everything". In my opinion this is vital, simply because we have a limited amount of time to develop these young people, so I want to make sure that we aren't going to have to constantly start over and repeat what we did. I hate repeating myself, so why would I want to do the same program in the fall that I did in the spring and summer. If we follow these simple charts we can move forward consistently. As we progress throughout the year and come to a pausing point. (i.e. when the kids go home) we, maybe, do a bit of work similar to where we left off to just give body a reminder of what we did in the summer. This idea is nothing new to our field. A quick couple weeks to jump start us back is way more efficient then repeating an entire 8-week block to regain the speed work that we lost over the 3-4 weeks of down time. At least it is in my opinion.

Why are we doing this?

The next thing we need to discuss is the goal of this program. The goal of this program is simple, to provide an adequate stimulus to make practice easier, while not taking away from the athlete's ability to continue to practice. Ok, let's unwrap this word salad a bit and into what this truly means.

First, let's talk about the last part because that's most important. We never, ever, want to take away from the athlete's ability to work on perfecting their craft. I don't care if you agree with what's being done on the court or not, that's what they're there for, so we have to do everything in our power to ensure that they're available to be able to perform this work at the highest level possible. So, with that in mind, we don't run here. We use this time to do off foot conditioning. You may ask "why?"; well two reasons. The first is that there is a history of basketball players having overuse issues with their knees, backs, ankles, and some groin problems. So, at this time of the year, if we can improve GENERAL aerobic qualities without putting greater stress on the joints that are typically "trouble" areas, we will remove that. Secondly, they're running at practice, on hard wood, in basketball shoes. That's enough pounding on their joints for me.

The next part is where it gets tricky. Providing an adequate stimulus that makes practice easier. What does that mean? Our goal is to improve the qualities that will allow the athlete to work at a higher level for a longer duration at practice. If they're able to increase the outputs at practice, and recover from them, then they should improve their outputs in games. Remember though, we cannot take away from the athlete's availability at practice. This is where it gets tricky because in basketball, when we say conditioning, coaches think about things like 16's and suicides with kids running to the garbage can to call for dinosaurs. And while I am not in the camp of never pushing the athletes into these "zones", I don't feel that the general phase is the time for this. There is 100% a time for it though, just not when we are working on general fitness. In this stage, we are going to work below the internal outputs of practice to help increase three things:

1. The intensity of the output before reaching "fatigue" states

2. The duration of work before reaching "fatigue" states

3. The athlete's ability to recover both within and between workouts

So, in a simpler sense, we want to increase the intensity and volume the athlete can work before fatigue sets in, and increase how quickly they can recover between reps/sets/segments of a practice, from practice to practice. And now for the best part, how we are going to do it, and why we make it optional.

Threshold Intervals

In what was the most unsexy programming decision I've made in my nearly 20 years as practitioner, using threshold intervals as our primary conditioning means in our general phase has been one that I truly believe has the greatest return on investment (ROI). When it comes down to it, this ticks a lot of boxes:

1. Inexpensive

2. Easily tracked to see improvement/when to make changes/progressive overload

3. Easily done "off feet"

4. Identify if athletes actually need to condition

With this year being how it's been keeping the price to a minimum is vital for all of us, but there are other ways to do this. So, within this section I'd like to share what we use, why we use it, it's limitations, and how you can probably do it better but we just can't yet.

Let's start with what we use. I ordered a bunch of H7 Polar heart rate monitors off Amazon. I picked those because they're less than 60 bucks a pop and pair with a phone's Bluetooth. I then sent the guys each a link to download Polar Beat in the app store. There are some pros and cons to this "system". Other than the price point the biggest pro is that you have color coded zones for where you want the athletes to train. For this situation you're going to try to get them to "dance on the orange/red line". This is an estimation of where anaerobic threshold (AnT) is. Before people start jumping up and down, yes, I know AnT isn't an actual thing, and that we produce lactate at all times, and that all our energy systems work in symphony, and that it's more an issue of hypoxia when the hydrogen ion is removed upon the lactic acid leaving the cell, and I understand that it is actually a local issue that may not be accurately determined by heart rate. I got it, I've said it, I've made all these arguments in the past, but it is the best we've got right now, and to be honest it seems to work pretty well. So even with all that, that's not the biggest issue with the system and this set up. To stay completely candid, I need to share that though. As Dr. Mann mentioned earlier in this book, these numbers are estimations, and even though you can change the max heart rate in the app, the "zones" are still a guess. Of course, I'd rather have the target ranges be more individualized and specific based off lactate tests or gas exchange (Think VO2 Max), but for the price it's a sacrifice I have to make at the present moment. Once we get a larger system for team use (which is in the works) we can input max heart rates for each individual and decrease the amount of inaccuracy. To find these max heart rates we will do some sort of max effort test (obviously this hasn't been established yet because at the time of writing this we aren't doing it) and we will then input that max heart rate into the system. This will change the numbers within the ranges so they are individualized for each athlete. (Note: for these tests though, they need to be task specific. So, if you're running, run, if you're using a Versaclimber, do that, but don't expect different modalities to elicit the same max heart rate, because simply, they won't.) For now, though, until I can track it in the system itself and not have to continue to go back into the athlete's phone to look at and adjust those numbers I'll deal with all those issues and stay with what we got because it seems to be working and the guys like it. So, to summarize, the strap and button is inexpensive and we are using a free app that allows us to say, "make the number go as high as it can and stay orange for this long." We are sacrificing some accuracy because I don't want to mess with their phones and keep going into the app to adjust the numbers to allow the guys to start to understand what we are going to ask them to be doing in the future as our technology improves. To start, we went simple, and simple seems to almost always be good.

Simple includes simple ways to see and track progress, and simple ways to identify when we need to make changes. For the above devices mentioned it's very simple. We perform the workout two times a week. Each time we record the distance covered per set. If we cover more distance, while staying in the same heart rate zone, for the same amount of time, we can then infer that we are improving. We can also look at what the recovery heart rates are between sets, and two minutes after completion of the workout, the latter being the most important. When the distance covered does not improve two workouts in a row, we then increase the work being done, either by adding a set or adding a minute per set. Progressive overload moving at the rate necessary based on how the athlete is showing us they're adapting. It really might be that simple.

The next point of importance is that it's easy to do off feet. We have four options for the teams to use: Versaclimber, concept2 ski erg, concept2 rower, and rogue echo bikes. Each of which has their own pros and cons and reasons why the kids would want to use them. Each of these also allow the heart rate sensor to connect to them as well (so they have a backup view of where they are) and have the ability to have the phone in the athlete's vision so they can see what their heart rate is at that moment to make sure they're in the "zones" required. The goal is always to keep the goal the goal, so these four have been picked because they allow athletes with unique injury histories to have options to pick what feels best for them. Honestly, I don't care which one they use, that's not the fight I'm going to pick. I want to make sure that, whichever it is, they are dialed in to what they're doing, track their improvement, and it doesn't increase/cause any pain that impacts their ability to practice.

The final point is probably the most important, and that is identifying if an athlete actually needs to follow this method. To be frank, not all athletes need to condition. I know, it's shocking to hear, but there is a vast array of reasons why an athlete wouldn't need to do extra conditioning. The easiest reason to identify is that they play all year round. Because of this year round play there are some athletes who have built a huge motor and a massive special work capacity. For those athlete's the juice might not be worth the squeeze, and you may be better off finding better uses of their time.

Prescription and Progression

Now for the gold at the end of my rambling rainbow. The way we utilize this method is really quite simple. We have three different "programs" that the guys follow.

The first is that this is their conditioning protocol. With this "group" they will come in two times a week, typically on the "nonlift days" (Tuesday and Thursday for this group). Week one of the program starts with six sets of 4 minutes in the "zone" and a minute break between sets (typically written 6(4:00/1:00). The first set is used as a warm up. We track the workout by looking at distance per set, total distance covered in the five working sets, and two-minute recovery heart rate. As long as those continue to improve, we continue with the same protocol, because we are making the assumption that if the athlete is improving in these then there is no need to do more (think minimal effective dose for your conditioning here, and exactly what Steffan talked about earlier in the book). When the athlete stalls for 2 workouts in a row we will add a set and see if the progress picks back up, which it typically does.

The second group is athletes that have one of two issues: 1) they do not have big enough drop, and therefore have a hard time recovering between bouts. This leads to them having huge drop offs in outputs, 2) have some body comp issues and we want them to do a little extra work to lean up a bit. In "old school" terms, they're not in shape. The plan for them is to perform the AnT work 2-3 times a week after practice on Monday, Wednesday, and/or Friday. The third day will be an optional session for them, but because these are done after practice we cut the sessions down and start at 4 sets at 4:00/1:00. On Tuesday and Thursday, in the place of the AnT work that group 1 is doing, these athletes will do 30:00-45:00 of steady state work on Tuesday and Thursday. These sessions are done on the same modality as their AnT work, and will be done in the "green zone". We will track total distance on these to make sure that the athlete is progressing with the training. Once they become stagnant and don't improve on the "green" work for 2 workouts in a row, we will add 5 minutes to the training, so they would start at 30:00 and progress to 35:00. The threshold work is progressed similarly to group one. Once that stalls for two workouts in a row we add a set. If we run into the situation where practice performance starts to plummet, we will take out one of the "green days" per week.

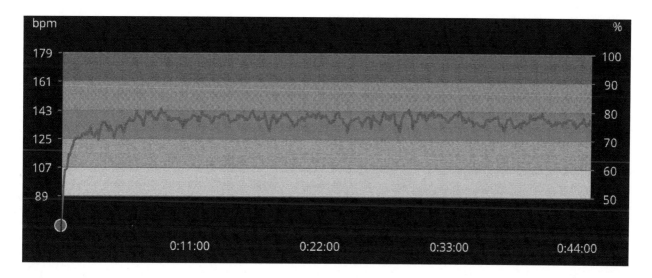

Example of "Green" Day

Remember, I mentioned above you could identify athletes who may not even need to perform this method? Well that's the third group. The players who just don't need to condition. There are so many reasons why you would exclude someone from doing extra conditioning. With that being said, I may have a way to look at their workout to see if they are "fit enough" if you will. To identify if this is even worthwhile for your athletes you look at the summary of the workout after and look at the heart rate drops in each set. There are four things that need to occur for them to be exempt:

1) Their heart rate between sets drops into the "blue" zone. This is somewhere in the area of a 40 beats per min drop in 60 seconds. That's pretty darn good.

2) If they can spike their heart rate fast. The "incline" should be as sharp as the decline. Otherwise they may be dogging it a bit earl on.

3) The athlete can get to the "red line" and "dance" there (+ or – 5 bpm) for the allotted duration of time.

4) Their two-minute recovery heart rate drops into the "grey" zone. This drop is going to be over 60 beats per minute in a two-minute span.

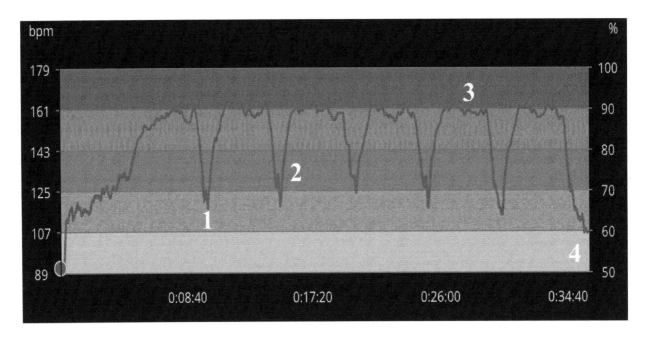

Example of "Fit Enough", so AnT work is optional

Once an athlete has ticked these boxes, they're plenty fit for the game of basketball. Can this quality improve? Of course it can. Is it the best use of the athlete's adaptive reserves when it comes to improving performance? That's a conversation between you and the athlete. Only you two can answer that.

Conclusion

Like everything I program, I'm sure that many people are thinking "is that really it?" The answer is, yes, yes that's it. As big of a numbers nerd as I am, and a technology geek as I tend to be, I keep coming back to simple methods that are have been tried and tested and shown to be successful. Andrew Althoff penned a chapter in Vol. 4 that was titled "Boring Stuff Works". He's 100% right. I would argue, though, that if you can display that there are positive results coming from the work, then that shouldn't be boring. I know I'm not alone in that thought process, but am not naive enough to think that no one is shaking their head at me right now as well. Unfortunately, positive results aren't enough for everyone, and for some the repetitive nature will be a bit dull. You may need to find ways to spice it up a bit. Even if it's as simple as rotating modalities to keep it fresh, that's fine. As long as you can chart progress and show the athletes that they're improving, and when/why it's time to make changes then they're improving and you're winning. The time when it's not ok though is when making it fun takes away from their ability to practice and improve sport form. Always remember, you're there to help them be better at the sport, not better at whatever machine they're doing their conditioning work on. So, the minute on court work starts to suffer, what's the first thing I cut? The thing you just read about for the last 11 pages!

Who is Jay DeMayo?

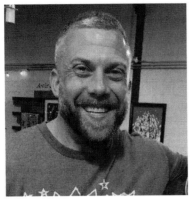

Jay DeMayo is in his 18th year as a strength and conditioning coach at the University of Richmond, and his 16th year working with the men's basketball team in 2019-20.

DeMayo is directly responsible for the strength training, conditioning and flexibility development of the men and basketball and tennis teams. He also educates the student-athletes on the proper nutrition to make sure their bodies are performing to their full potential.

In conjunction with his role with the Spiders, Jay also is the head of dry land training for NOVA Aquatics, LLC where he has worked with multiple Olympic trial qualifiers and 2016 Olympic Gold Medalist Townley Haas.

If that wasn't enough, Jay also is the owner of Central Virginia Sport Performance, a coaching education company most known from their three weekly podcasts (My Thoughts Monday, Outside the Rack, and The Podcast) and their yearly symposium, The Seminar. CVASPS also has published 5 books (The Manual, Vol. 1-5...well 6 now if you're reading this) as well.

As a top expert in field of strength and nutrition, DeMayo has presented at dozens of seminars and clinics across the country. He has also coached and lectured for a month at Ningbo University in China.

DeMayo came to Richmond from Indiana State, where he was a graduate assistant during the 2002-03 academic year. The Fairport, N.Y. native played on the soccer team at SUNY-Cortland.

10

A Complete Change in Coaching Philosophy; From Control to Autonomy

And Why I'm Never Going Back

Ali Kershner

I vividly remember sitting alone on my couch, peak COVID shutdown, aimlessly scrolling through the pages of the excel template I had just finished writing. It felt like Phase 87 of a never-ending micro-cycle. Mid scroll, a sinking feeling set in – unable to see or talk to my athletes (let alone coach them), I knew that beautifully manicured workout card probably meant next to nothing.

I started to wonder if that feeling was due to me missing my job or to an all-consuming worry that I hadn't prepared my athletes in a way that would ensure they could successfully execute the program without me there to monitor it.

Had I taught them enough to perform the workouts safely on their own?

Had I empowered them to self-select alternatives when one didn't feel good?

Had they learned to make smart decisions about when to push and when to pull back?

Had they learned anything at all from me?

Okay that last one was a bit melodramatic but I was in my head at that point. Either way, these questions prompted one more –

Going forward, if my athletes were to gain just ONE thing from working with me, what would I want it to be?

1. Improve overall strength, conditioning, and health?

2. Become more efficient and effective in their sport?

3. Buy-in to the benefit of the weight room?

4. Build resilience by enduring adversity and discomfort?

5. Take ownership in their improvement/learn skills they will use for the rest of their lives

My real answer is #5, but all that time I had been acting as if it was #1...

Armed with a clarified purpose, I spent the next several weeks evaluating whether my programming and coaching style was reflecting that desired goal.

The result? Not even close.

Let's look at this from a macro-level and then narrow in.

The typical collegiate athlete is over scheduled, plain and simple. They seldom have time to make decisions or exercise creativity when every minute of their day is planned for them. For example, a typical routine might look something like this: morning lift, straight to breakfast, class, lunch, treatment, practice, class, dinner, bed.

Not only that – at the places I've coached even during the activity where you'd think they could experiment and exercise creativity (read: practice), they are in many ways stymied through structure.

Now going deeper, I certainly didn't help the situation. My type-A self, enjoyed presenting a perfectly formatted, crisp workout card. I found peace in a scientifically sound annual program with elaborate periodization and I took pride in having my lifts look and run like a well-oiled machine. In essence I had been contributing to this controlled system and treating my athletes like robots: Rinse, Lather, Repeat.

I had been over-programming and over-coaching because _I controlled what I didn't trust_.

Humbled by this realization, I set out in search of ways to create a learning environment.

I knew of coaches that used autonomy and choice as a coaching philosophy but I had always dismissed it as an appropriate method for an exceptionally motivated team or a hands-off coach, but not me.

Reading _Drive_ by Daniel Pink and diving more into the concept of Self-Determination Theory was the start of a turning point. I finally began to understand that we (humans) are motivated most when fueled by autonomy, competence, and relatedness.

This makes sense. I never wanted to learn how to change a tire until I was out on the side of the road with a blowout. I had no interest in balancing a checkbook or managing finances until I lived on my own making a graduate assistant salary. The reality is many of us don't learn until we have to. If we can rely on someone else telling us how or doing it for us, why would we purposefully induce extra cognitive load? Evolutionarily it doesn't make sense.

The same is true of training. Few of our athletes inherently LOVE the weight room. Rather – (if we're lucky) they see it as a means to an end. But taking care of their body and knowing how to exercise safely is a skillset that will serve them far beyond sport.

With this in my mind, I decided to utilize autonomy and choice as primary tenets in my programming so long as we were lucky enough to return post COVID. Besides, in addition to stimulating motivation and learning, there are a plethora of advantages to creating an autonomous environment for both coach and athlete. If done correctly (or even semi-correctly), there's a high likelihood they will:

1. Gain a sense of ownership in their program

2. Develop the skill of "figuring it out" and rely less on constant feedback

3. Begin to understand what feels "good" and what doesn't

4. Learn general programming principles

5. Buy-in to you as a coach and see that you care about them

6. Individualize the program to fit personal physiological and psychological needs

7. Lift objectively heavier loads with higher intensities

8. Have higher satisfaction with their performance in the weight room

9. Auto-regulate when fatigued and/or overreached

10. Generate fewer excuses (I mean; it was *their* choice…)

11. Understand the importance of and what goes into creating a high functioning body

12. do you really need more reasons??

Okay, but how does one go from complete control to absolute autonomy?

In my mind, I pictured a coach walking into the weight room on Day 1, throwing workout cards into the air and declaring a free for all... An image probably as scary as realizing your athletes haven't learned anything.

Personally, I worried that my players would see me as a fraud for undergoing a complete reconstruction of my coaching philosophy after just one year. Again, questions swirled and insecurities bubbled to the surface:

Did I even know what I was talking about?

Would I be able to relinquish control and allow them a safe place to fail?

What if my head coach walked in and saw the messy and imperfect reps- would I lose credibility?

What if it didn't work?

I say all this to remind you, the reader, that before I could do a deep dive on the methodology and structure of an autonomy-based program (now there's an oxymoron), I had to do some serious work on myself. I knew the athletes would handle it just fine, but would I?

Once I came to the realization that the risk was worth the reward, I set out to interview coaches who programmed like this and research how one actually makes this transition.

Surprise, surprise – it's not as thrilling as my mind made it out to be...

Here's what I found and here's how I implemented it in my program. Heads up – it requires work up front, a ramp up period and progressive overload *Cough, like everything else in sports performance, *cough, cough*:

1. **Lay the ground rules and tell them why**

   On day 1, I gathered my group together, explained the reasons for giving them more autonomy in the weight room, the benefits of doing so and why learning sound exercise technique would be important not only for today, but 10 years from now.

2. **Use your GPP phase to introduce variety**

The key to autonomy is to actually have options they can pick from. If you've only ever taught them one variation of a squat and one variation of a pull, there's no choice! The GPP phase is inherently a teaching block so throw in different variations of every movement to expand their "exercise bank".

3. **Give them an exercise bank to remind them what they know**

Even we as coaches forget all of the different variations we know. Keep track of what they've learned and let them refer back to the list so they don't get stuck doing the same thing over and over.

4. **Micro-dose choice**

If you do nothing else, DO THIS – I can't stress it enough. Start with tiny amounts of choice and build up. None of my programs are completely autonomous. One way to start is to make the warm-up "choice based" (Appendix B). Utilize games to get them used to making decisions and being creative from the jump then introduce choice in small quantities throughout the workout. For example, maybe they pick the mobility or core exercise paired with the main lift. Finally, ramp up opportunities for choice slowly - one workout isn't enough to get them adjusted.

5. **Provide guardrails by categorizing movements or creating "buckets"**

I'd list the type of movement and then let them decide within that category. For example, one training block would look like this:

A1. Bilateral Squat: (Choice – Safety Bar, Trap Bar, Back, Front, Pit Shark)

A2. Bilateral Upper Pull: (Choice - Supported Row, Power Stance Row, Inverted Row, Bent Over Row)

A3. Rotational Core: (Choice - Down Chop, Cable Trunk Rotation, MB L-Over, MB Rotational Throw)

I've included an example of our lifts from this year and some of the warm-ups I've used in the past to help promote autonomy at the end. DON'T SKIP AHEAD (Appendix A)

6. **Keep reiterating the purpose**

I'd remind them of the points discussed in #1 several times. When they'd tell me they didn't want to choose, I'd remind them of the importance of autonomy (learning) and then help them select one that felt good to them.

7. **Encourage choice, novelty & mistakes**

THIS IS SO IMPORTANT. It's not going to look great, in fact sometimes you might look out on the floor and be embarrassed by what you see. Look, having 15 different programs happening at once is going to drive you crazy as a coach and it's going to be difficult to not correct mistakes. Let them happen- it's the only way learning occurs. If it feels out of hand, scale back on the autonomy a little bit, regress certain movements within the movement bank but PLEASE, don't take away choice just because it doesn't look clean...

8. **Don't over-program choice**

This is an interesting and important one. Not everyone is going to love choice. In fact, I'd be willing to bet some of your athletes will be very resistant to it. Remember, it's a cognitive load and some people just want to be told what to do. They don't want the responsibility of doing it themselves and that's okay. It will take a little more time and education on your part but it doesn't mean they won't come around. Micro-dose their choice slower and smaller. Help them make decisions and then let the reins out slowly. Once they have a feel for how empowering it is to pick what they like, they will come around. Also remember how much else they have going on in their life. Some athletes come to the weight room and want to check out mentally, grind, and sweat. There are times and places for that but there are also long-term benefits to this. Expose them to both.

That's it: Educate on the front end, ramp up slowly, micro-dose the amount of choice, and be okay with imperfection.

After telling people about my experience coaching with autonomy, I usually get asked "how do you know it worked"

Simple.

One day, one of my basketball players walked up to me and said, "Can you remind me of the single leg squat options- I think I'm ready to progress to something harder..."

After running down the list of single leg squat variations we had learned, she turned to me and said, "Can I make one up?"

Not sure whether to be impressed, proud, or surprised, I nodded.

She proceeded to set up a single leg squat stand facing a rack. She attached a band to the rack and looped it around the back of her knee as if to do a TKE (terminal knee extension). She then grabbed dumbbells and proceeded to descend into her single leg squat.

After a few reps she turned to me and said, "I really like the way the band forces me to engage my quad at the top of the movement, I feel it a lot more."

At that moment, I wanted to drop a mic and walk out of the weight room. Instead, as the poised individual I am, I told her "Great work! I'm naming that after you," and went to help the next athlete.

Hindsight is 20/20 but now I truly can't imagine doing it any other way.

Given the year we had – 10 weeks (straight) on the road, lifting primarily outside and in hotel weight rooms - trying to implement my old programming style within these constraints would have been impossible... In fact, the only way we were able to embrace the chaos and thrive in the uncertainty was by leaning on a foundation of choice.

Now I'd be remiss if I told you autonomy is the greatest thing since sliced bread and should be adopted by everyone immediately. Nowhere close. In fact, there are aspects I question every day - specifically, what's causing what? It's hard to tell when programming isn't linear and there isn't a clear line between A and B.

And there are other factors to consider... For example, would I use autonomy all year long? Not to the extent I do during the season. There are times when programs need more direction and constraint. There are times when education and technique need to be specified- especially at the front end and with novice athletes.

Would I say it's appropriate for every team and coach? NO! Definitely not. Again, it's about fit. Know your context, decide what your goals are and find a solution to bridge the two. This was mine.

I'll end by saying this-

If you want to create a true learning environment choice and failure are essential ingredients. Autonomy is but one way to accomplish that.

Appendix A:

Sample Week of In-Season Lifts

The following two workouts are an example of a week of in-season training for us. The column on the left "written on the board" indicates what I had programmed. The column on the right illustrates what one athlete ended up picking. Remember- this was different for literally every athlete on the floor and this was a program I used toward the end of the season when autonomy had become a regular practice. Earlier in the season, I would have specified a few more movements giving them slightly less autonomy than you see below.

Another note: I didn't give them a choice in the sets and reps. That might be something to experiment with in the future but we weren't ready for that just yet...

Not pictured: The exercise bank with different variations we'd learned. Once they got better at this, I'd verbally remind them of options but wouldn't have to list them out.

Day 1: Lower Focus

	Written on the board	What one athlete picked:	Sets x Reps
A1.	Lower Plyo	KB Swing	3 x 10
A2.	Mobility / Stretch	Shinbox Twist (90/90 position)	3 x 5e
B1.	Bilateral Squat	Front Squat	5/3/2/2/2/2
B2.	Unilateral Upper Push	1 Arm Landmine Shoulder Press	4 x 5e
C1.	Unilateral Hinge	Single Leg DB RDL	3 x 5e
C2.	Bilateral Upper Pull	Pull-up	3 x 2
C3.	Core (Anti-Rotational)	Loaded Plank	3 x 20s

Day 2: Upper Focus

	Written on the board	What one athlete picked:	Sets x Reps
A1.	Upper Plyo	MB Linear Slam	3 x 6
A2.	Mobility / Stretch	Thoracic Rotation	3 x 5e
B1.	Bilateral Upper Push	Incline DB Chest Press	4 x 5
B2.	Unilateral Squat	RFE Split Squat	4 x 5e
C1.	Unilateral Pull	1 Arm KB Supported Row	3 x 5e
C2.	Bilateral Hinge	BB Hip Lift	3 x 5
C3.	Core (Rotational)	Cable Trunk Rotation	3 x 5e

Appendix B:

Autonomy Warm-up Activities

1. **Design Your Own Warm-Up:**

Instructions: Pick one from each category. 5-10 reps per movement x 3 rounds. Categories: Intrinsic foot exercise, favorite stretch, favorite mobility exercise, body weight squat variation, push-up variation, snap down.

2. **Interact with a KB:**

Instructions: Pick up a 12kg KB. Carry, Squat, Row, Press, Anything - just don't put it down for 5 mins.

3. **Obstacle Course:**

Instructions: Set up implements that the athlete has to interact with. Example: physioball, foam roller, Airex Pad, ladder, plyo box, etc. Have them move from a specified point A to point B interacting in a different way with each implement laid out.

4. **Mirror Your Partner:**

Instructions: Set up 2 cones 10y apart. Athletes stand on opposite sides of the cones as if the line between the cones was an invisible fence between the two. One athlete begins moving between the two cones, skipping, stretching, hopping, running, etc. The other athlete has to mirror them. Do 30s intervals and switch a few times.

Who is Ali Kershner?

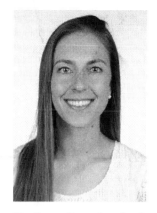

Ali Kershner is The Director of Creative Strategy for Art of Coaching where she works on all aspects of live events, mentorship, creative content and marketing. Prior to joining Art of Coaching, Ali was the Associate Sports Performance Coach for Stanford Women's Basketball and Women's Golf from 2019-2021. While at Stanford, she helped the Cardinal to a PAC-12 Title and National Championship.

Before Stanford, she was an Assistant Sports Performance Coach at Kansas from 2017-2019 and spent the two years prior to that as a graduate assistant in the department. In her position she primarily worked with the women's soccer, women's basketball, swimming and women's golf teams.

Originally from Palo Alto, California, Ali graduated from Duke in 2015 with a bachelor's degree in evolutionary anthropology. While in Durham she spent four highly-successful seasons as a member of the soccer team. A captain and goalkeeper for the Blue Devils, Ali and her Duke teams advanced to the Elite Eight three times and made the College Cup final in 2011.

Ali earned her master's in exercise physiology from Kansas in 2017. She is a certified strength and conditioning specialist by the National Strength and Conditioning Association.

Made in the USA
Middletown, DE
18 July 2021